Second printing 2017

First published by Backfitpro Inc..

150 Evans Ave W.,
Gravenhurst, Ontario, Canada P1P 1A8

www.backfitpro.com

ISBN: 978-0-9735018-2-7

This book is printed on acid-free paper

Printed in Canada

Cover design by Paal Hawk, for Altius Gruppen AS, Hamar, Norway.
Photographer: Lars A. Lien
Model: A. Haglund
All drawings by Jiri Hvalacek, Prague, Czech Republic.

Acknowledgements

This is my third book. Instead of getting easier, the process was more difficult. The challenge lay in getting the book as small as possible while incorporating the details necessary for people to rid their back of pain. This constant conflict and analysis is hardest on the people who are closest to me. My wife Kathryn bears the brunt of it. Like most husbands, I am a work in progress. All I can say is I am better today than yesterday, and will strive to be better tomorrow.

The team was truly international. The wonderful illustrations were created by the very talented Jiri Hlavacek of Prague, Czech Republic. His images conveyed the postures and movements with crystal clarity. The cover design was the brainchild of Paal Hawk, a gifted graphic designer in Hamar, Norway. Truth be known, I had two editors review my manuscript but neither reflected my voice. It is difficult to remove my medical jargon and replace it with common everyday language. I need help with this. I was working in Los Angeles and I opened an email from my son John who now resides in New York City, USA. The email message read, "Dad, saw your manuscript on the kitchen table. I read the first chapter and re-wrote it. What do you think?" Tears came to my eyes in that hotel room. What I had been looking for was under my nose all the time. Thank you son.

The material contained in this book has a strong foundation in the science produced in our lab/clinic. I must acknowledge the -40plus graduate students and visiting scholars who have contributed to building that foundation. I must thank the patients who have attended our University clinic for back pain consults, and who taught us much wisdom. Finally, I thank you the reader, who have asked me to write this book for years. Thank you all.

Table of Contents

Getting the Most out of this Book

If we're going to liken the spine to a vehicle and the author to a mechanic, then consider this book to be the manual. This will be your definitive text when it comes to learning how to diagnose your own back conditions, and identify the best recovery plan suited to you. Unlike a car manual, however, I suggest you read this book cover to cover as opposed to rapidly flipping the pages trying to find a paragraph or two that applies to you. The truth is this, if you are a back pain sufferer, this whole book applies to you! Unlike a car where changing out one part can cure the problem, back pain is more complicated as the problem is usually in more than a single part. As you begin to draw some conclusions about your specific spinal circumstances, you may come across the occasional section that does not apply to you and you will skip, but in general I would recommend reading through the entire progression from A to Z. The broader your understanding, the greater your success.

To maximize your retention and effective application of this text, I would even recommend reading this book through twice! The first time, mentally digest the information and take notes on tips that you find particularly helpful or ideas you have about incorporating the recommendations into your daily life. For the second pass through, get physical! Put on loose clothing, clear an area in your house, and follow the diagnostic tests and rehabilitative exercises in real time as you read! This twice-through system is especially important during the self-diagnosis found in Section II.

As you progress, you will come across two types of "breakout" sections. Let's take a moment to familiarize ourselves with those.

Patient Files: In these sections we will examine the stories of real-life patients I've had and discuss the tips and tricks they discovered on their individual roads to recovery. Although their names have been changed for confidentiality purposes, each of these individuals came through my office at some point in the last three decades. Just like them, you will soon have your own recovery story to tell.

Insights from the Podium: Over the course of my career, I've had the opportunity to work with athletes on many levels, from high school competitors to professional teams to Olympic gold medalists. These breakouts will provide quotes and wisdom from the champions I've worked with in a wide array of athletic disciplines. True, we may not all be looking to hold world records, but these individuals have overcome back trouble while pushing their bodies to their limits as part of their careers. Their wisdom, coming from an extreme level of physicality, can transcend to anyone looking to better their spine health.

It is important to know that although many physicians are familiar with my work, some are not. If you continue to seek professional care during or after your completion of this text, I encourage you to bring this book with you to consultations so that you and your physician are both on the same page about your current course of recovery.

Additionally, if, after reading this book, you find that you want to delve deeper into literature on back health, and are curious to read more about my research lab and our findings, I invite you to read my other published books. The first is titled *Low Back Disorders*, and the second, *Ultimate Back Fitness and Performance*. If your goal is simply to understand and address your own personal back pain so that you can get back to the activities you always loved, look no further. I have every confidence that at the end this book, you will feel as though I've passed along the role of back mechanic from me the author, to you the reader.

Professor Stuart McGill,
Waterloo, Canada

Introduction

The Secrets to a Healthy Spine Your Doctor Isn't Telling You

You may be wondering what sets this book apart. Why out of the multitude of back books available is this the one that will make a difference in your life. The truth is simple: the information contained in this book comes down to cold hard science. Eliminating back pain is not simple. I was strongly encouraged to write a book entitled "5 Easy Steps to eliminating back pain" or something similar to gain mass appeal. This has no integrity, nor truth. I will guide you, and in return I need your commitment to follow the details in this book.

From my early work in spine biomechanics as a PhD student over thirty years ago, to the revolutionary discoveries made in my lab/clinic at the University of Waterloo, I have established a reputation that draws patients to visit from around the world, together with doctors and scientists requesting guidance. I was using motion capture technology long before the producers of the film "Avatar," in conjunction with monitoring the biophysical signals of the body to determine how it works, as well as how it becomes pained. My team employs many approaches including working on real spines from cadavers to decipher injury mechanisms, working on pained people to uncover the cause of their pain, performing group studies to find out what is effective, and routinely working with some of the world's top athletes, from the UFC, NHL, NBA, NFL professional leagues, powerlifting federations, the adventure sports, and dozens of Olympic athletes. These multiple approaches assist in discovering better ways to regain lost physical abilities. Why work with athletes? Driving a Ferrari teaches you what is possible with elite automotive technology and skill. Our discoveries enabled us to heal quite massive spine damage so completely that some athletes returned to set another world record. This is proof that cannot be dismissed.

Many have asked me to write a version of my textbooks that would be easily consumable by the lay public. Being successful in rebuilding backs is not easy, nor is it easy to simplify. But here it is. I have taken all of my discoveries from the years and boiled them down into the facts, the straight truth about back pain, the cause, and the programs that work to fix it. I have no political agenda, no medical associations, no drug companies or surgical appliance companies, no governments to appease. You will find in this book the truth you've been looking for, the instructions you wish your family doctor had given you, and the science you wish the specialist had been armed with before he told you that surgery was your only option.

Too often, medical "professionals" are quick to dismiss back pain, saying the "discomfort in your lower back is of no known origin," or "it's all in your head," or "you have little chance of improvement, here's some painkillers…" Sound familiar? I'm here to tell you that you have seen an individual who is giving advice beyond their level of competency and expertise. I hear about misguided advice like this from patients on a daily basis and they come back to me weeks after being on my program with an absolute turn around. 95% of you will benefit, I know this because we follow up with our patients.

Within the pages of this book you will find your step by step guide to getting your spine back in top condition. You will learn:

1. The distinct causes and progressions of back pain, from disc bulges to sciatica.
2. The potential activities in your daily schedule that are causing and aggravating back pain.
3. Healthy movement patterns that will promote pain-free living, and allow you to continue to do the activities you always loved.
4. Strategies and exercises to help you achieve and maintain a healthy and robust spine.
5. The mandatory checklist items for whether surgery will help or make the situation worse.

This book is for everyone who wants their swagger back, from the homemaker who misses the spring in her step and wants to be able to walk the dog free of pain, to the former NFL player who is so plagued by chronic back pain that he can barely find the will to get out of bed. I've dealt with both types of patients first hand and after reading this book you will understand the science behind my high success rate with patients and be able to apply these techniques yourself.

You deserve to get down on the floor and play with the kids with the ease of movement you used to have. Isn't it a basic human necessity to be able to sleep through the night without waking yourself up with excruciating pain every time you roll over? Living with your current situation is not much fun. It's not going to be easy. Getting your spine in working order is going to take discipline and commitment. You're going to have to break old habits and form some new ones. But you owe it to yourself to know what it's like to make it through the day free of pain and discomfort. It's time to take charge of your life again. It's time to start fresh and give your spine an overhaul. It's time to get your swagger back.

Let's begin.

Part One:
"Why me?" Understanding your pain

Chapter 1 examines the wisdoms and notions that you have heard about your back pain. What is true and what should you believe? Chapter 2 introduces you to your back, how the various parts work, and what causes pain. The order in which you choose to read these two chapters depends on your learning style. If you are more curious as to why the previous approaches have not worked for you when they helped a friend, then read chapter 1 first. If you desire insight into how your back works, read chapter 2 first.

Chapter 1

Mythbusting

Mythbusting

In these first two chapters, I'm going to make sure we're on the same page in terms of what the spine really is and how it functions, and sort out the fact from the fiction by dispelling some common myths surrounding our backs. Unfortunately, you have been subjected to many myths and no doubt these have led you to your painful condition. It is only by working from the ground up, and establishing this basic knowledge that we can then move forward in learning how to assess and rehabilitate ourselves.

During an appointment for back pain, many physicians will spend far too short a time with the patient, who often comes away with no diagnosis at all or else a very specific conclusion that was reached merely by looking at the MRI or CT image. In my opinion, this is already a failed exam. Determining someone's source of pain from glancing over such a picture is like looking at a visual of a car, with no other information and determining the reason that the engine won't start. Even when a diagnosis is reached, such as sciatica or a disc bulge, this assessment is hardly helpful in guiding the patient to a cure. One of the most important things you should glean from this book is that instead of focusing on the title of your condition, we must turn our attention to finding the cause of the symptoms and addressing them directly as a means to recovery.

Rather than centering its efforts on this philosophy, the medical community continues to focus its efforts on surgery recommendations as a "quick-fix" solution as well as pain relief in pill form as a means of sweeping the issue under the rug, so to speak. Myths and falsehoods arise in lieu of diagnosing an adequate and accurate cause of pain. For example, there are some experts and books out there making the claim that most pain "is all in your head." Pain almost always has a physical cause. Ignoring it or blaming it on yourself will get you no relief. I caution the seeking of psychotherapy as treatment for your back pain! Psychosocial issues, such as whether or not an individual likes their job, or whether or not a patient is neurotic, can modulate pain but these are not the original cause. Even if your doctor claims not to be able to determine the cause: be assured there is one, and it can be addressed.

The other persistent myth is that you will get used to your back pain, that it is something to which eventually you will grow accustomed and that your pain will decrease in sensitivity over time. Wrong! The truth is, the longer you go without addressing the pain, the more pain you perceive and the more sensitive you will become to it. Consider this analogy: If I were to hit my thumb repeatedly with a hammer, I sensitize my thumb; making it more sensitive to pain. Eventually, I will sensitize the tissue to the point that even the lightest touch, such as simply brushing my hand against my pants as I reach into my pocket causes me to wince with pain. In this case exercise will not be beneficial, but removing the hammer will. The first step to recovery we will deal with in this book is removing those "pain-hammers." You will show yourself that it is possible to replace painful activities with pain-free movements. This is the real solution to dialing down pain sensitivity as it will allow you to gradually expand your repertoire of activities you can enjoy pain-free.

It's a shame that when the truth is so shrouded in mythology and misinformation, the real people that suffer are the patients themselves. Their recovery is hindered and their experience with past therapy has reinforced their belief that nothing can reduce their pain except surgery. This often leaves them deeply fearful, hardly comforted by the stories from friends who now rely on narcotic pain relievers just to make it through the day. They often feel hopeless and resign themselves to the idea that they will never be pain free.

It's time to sort the fact from the fiction, and establish some facts, attitudes, approaches and perspectives to demystify the pain and provide insight into the previous failure to properly address your back trouble.

Common Roadblocks

Let's begin with identifying some roadblocks, or personal barriers we create in our minds to recovery, and identify possible "detours" or suggestions for overcoming them on the road to the final destination of pain-free living:

Roadblock: My pain worsened after trying physical therapy.

Detour: It's time to find a physical therapist that understands and directly addresses the cause of your pain. Most likely you will be able to do this on your own guided by this book.

Roadblock: Every time I work out, I pay for it for the next three days.

Detour: By examining the components of the training session, your pain triggers and your activities throughout the other twenty-three hours of the day, it is likely we can find a correlation. We can then "tune" the aggravating activities to reduce your pain. More specific instructions on this later.

Roadblock: I've been told the pain is in my head.

Detour: Prove to yourself that you have the ability to enjoy some pain-free moments. This book will show you how to expand those moments into long-lasting relief.

Roadblock: I've been told I just have to be positive.

Detour: While being positive is a good suggestion, it is hardly ever effective when used as the only tool for pain reduction. Focus your efforts on determining and eliminating the cause of your pain.

Roadblock: I was advised by a clinic to record my pain on a scale of 1 to 10.

Detour: Direct your attention instead to discovering and enjoying pain free activity. Please disregard the workbook you have been given to "record" your pain levels.

Separating Fact from Fiction

We've already addressed two of the major myths circulating about back pain, both that it only exists in your head, and that it will eventually desensitize over time. Let's take a look at some more fiction and set the record straight.

Myth: *If my chronic back pain was not cured by following my physical therapist's guidance, surgery is my last remaining option.*

Fact: Have you ever heard the phrase "When all you have is a hammer, everything looks like a nail"? Most surgeons' come from the perspective that everything can be cured with a scalpel, if only you give him the opportunity to "cut the pain out." Rarely is the tissue that is being targeted for removal the only cause of the pain. Tissues that are in fact healthy, are often severed and destroyed when cutting down to reach the spine during surgery. The situation worsens when on occasion a nerve is severed in the process, compromising future rehabilitation. Furthermore, any metal hardware that is added to the spine during surgery can cause the local bone to weaken and the hardware to loosen. The risks associated with surgery often do not outweigh the potential benefits when we are dealing with cases in which the original source of pain is not being addressed. In these cases, the patient will often return within a couple years with similar tissue damage either above or below the previous site of surgery. Sometimes the original pain will reappear, only worse. Too often the surgeon will respond to these results with "There is nothing more I can do for you." With many of these patients, I have been able to provide solutions through rehabilitative exercises that target the pain source, but with some, the aftermath of the surgery has left them so intensely disabled that they are beyond my care. By reading this book, you are taking excellent steps towards exploring avenues that do not involve surgery, before resigning yourself to that option. The next chapter deals with the decision to undergo surgery and how to determine if and when this truly is the last remaining option.

Myth: The clinicians at the Pain Clinic will be able to provide me with a long-term solution.

Truth: Pain Management is exactly what it sounds like: management. It deals with the symptoms instead of addressing and alleviating the original cause. Because pain is a neural perception registered in the brain, a solution provided by a pain clinic will provide pills and cognitive based therapy. Typically a patient will be given heavy-duty pain medications that are highly addictive. This too is a common story I see with patients in which the medical system has failed them by masking the pain with drugs and neglecting the actual issue at hand.

Patient Files: Brad had become heavily addicted to the point of dependency to his pain killers. He had been prescribed them by a pain clinic after a doctor was unable to help him with his back and had left him with the classic misdiagnosis that it was "all in his head." He had also been advised to get a foot amputation because of the pain he was experiencing in one of his feet. Brad came to me admittedly suicidal, stating if he had truly invented this debilitating pain in his head then he must be crazy and didn't deserve to live. He told me we had a week to work together and alleviate his pain or he would kill himself. Talk about pressure. I worked closely with him over the following week and was able to show him that his condition was treatable. As it turned out, his feet were perfectly healthy and the pain he was experiencing was the result of a nerve trap in his lower back. We addressed this through avoidance of spine-flexing movement patterns and the increased fitness of the muscles responsible for controlling this motion. Over the next three months, as he overcame his dependency on the opiate pain killers and addressed his back condition directly, he was able to regain control of his life. Today he is quite happy and enjoys the full function of his back together with the foot a surgeon was so eager to remove.

Myth: Backs can be rehabilitated in 6-12 weeks. The length of insurance company payouts is clear evidence of this.

Fact: The studies cited by insurance companies in order to dictate this recovery period were actually conducted on muscle damage obtained from rodents. Studies conducted on human back injury contrarily show that, depending on the damage, there is often an extensive set of measures that must be taken in recovery and that true healing can take up to 10 years. This does not mean you must commit yourself to another 10 years of back pain – but it does mean that you will need to manage the way you load your back over a longer period of time in order to remain pain-free.

Myth: Back pain is always hereditary. My mother had back pain as long as I can remember – I am to expect the same thing.

Fact: Back pain is not a life sentence, nor a destiny. Although genetics may make certain individuals more susceptible to back issues than others, this is something that can be treated, and in most cases, avoided altogether. Many people believe that their back pain will only worsen as they age. Interestingly, most people have less pain around the age of retirement and they find they have grown out of it. They report that they experienced their worst symptoms during their thirties and forties. Nature gristled their back joints to reduce painful micromovements. How many older people complain about back pain? The fact is that very few do. To make sure you're not one of them, take the steps to manage and eliminate your pain now.

Myth: A herniated disc spells the end of a person's athletic career.

Fact: It is true that a damaged disk's recovery is far more uncertain and tricky than dealing with say, a fractured leg. Many athletes consider spine problems as the last injury they would ever want to deal with, but ultimately, with the right recovery program, these issues can be dealt with. I often work with elite athletes from a wide array of different sports. I have had hundreds return to successful careers in professional sports and the Olympics. Many of them have cleverly come up with their own systems to manage their problematic backs, even through the strains and stresses they place on their own bodies when training and competing. In working with these athletes as patients, I was able to give them a new set of tools to rehabilitate their damaged discs and get them back in the game and able to compete once again at their top performance level.

Insights from the Podium: One record setting Olympic weightlifter shared with me the story of how he had never set a world record prior to his back injury. He now holds three. The injuries became his "teacher" and provided him with some valuable insight he shared with me.

"In a way my back injuries were a blessing – the injuries forced me to adopt absolutely perfect technique: I could never again train with flawed or compromised form. Well, I could, but it would end my career once and for all."

When this world record holder started to train again he vowed to never break his "compromised technique" rule. His performance skyrocketed and he proceeded to reset his own world record two more times. Instead of being forced into retirement by an injury, he used it as fuel to refocus and "up" his game.

Myth: My MRI will provide the doctor with all he needs to know in terms of my course of treatment.

Truth: MRI and CT scan images are very limited in what they are able to tell us about causes of back pain. These "pictures" of your back will show changes and features that may or may not be the source of your pain. The pain source most usually stems from a functional issue. Flawed movement patterns, repeated over and over, sensitize your back tissues and drive them to be painful even when under very low load.

I cannot support an institute that looks solely at MRI and/ or CT images as the determining factor of whether or not you need surgery. These types of assessments must be conducted in person with a physician who has done homework in assessing and treating back conditions through pain provocation. These images can in fact prove useful once surgery has been determined to be the only remaining option (which is rare). They must be seen as simply one piece of evidence used in building the case for your optimal recovery plan.

Myth: Back pain is linked to having tight hamstrings.

Truth: Our research has found that in most cases, tight hamstrings are a related symptom of back issues rather than a cause. Interestingly, hamstrings often decrease in tightness as back pain subsides. That being said, when one hamstring is tighter than the other, the asymmetry has had mild influences on back pain, particularly in athletes. This book will teach you proper movement patterns for daily activities such as tying your shoes. You will learn that even those of you with tight hamstrings are able to perform such activities while sparing your back.

Myth: The darkly shaded disc on my MRI indicates I have "degenerative disc disease."

Truth: In the vast majority of cases, "degenerative disc disease" is a misdiagnosis. Dark shading of the discs visible on an MRI or CT scan is a sign of loss of water content in the spine. This happens to all of us as we age and is akin to the appearance of wrinkles on our faces. The idea of labeling this a "degenerative disease" is unnecessarily dramatic and is unhelpful in determining a course of action for the patient. However, if only one disc is different than the others in its apparent darkness, it is likely that it is a flattened disc and is the product of an injury – not aging. When left alone, (and not contorted into unnatural positions such as in yoga) this disc eventually stiffens over time and the pain resolves. As this natural healing process is occurring, the disc will naturally appear darker on an MRI.

Myth: Lying in bed is good for back pain.

Truth: In reality, lying in bed for excessive periods actually *causes* back pain. Let's examine this more closely. A little known fact is that we are all actually taller first thing in the morning than we are before we go to bed at night. This comes down to our discs. The discs in between each of our vertebrae are packed with very concentrated protein chains that love water. In scientific terms, this means they are "hydrophilic." When we lie horizontally, the discs fill with fluid and gently push the vertebrae away from one another, lengthening the spine. The reason, our backs are often stiff in the morning is that the discs are so full of fluid, like water balloons ready to burst. When we get up in the morning, and our spines are once again vertical, the excess of fluid in each disc begins to seep out and an hour or two after rising from bed we have returned to our normal heights. This natural ebb and flow is healthy and is what allows the discs to obtain nutrition. Problems arise, however, when the spine remains in a horizontal position for too long. While about eight hours in bed is healthy, much longer than that is not as it allows the spine to continue to swell and cause disc pain. Limiting your time in bed can help with this, as can selecting the right mattress for your back. More on this later.

Myth: My daily workouts at the gym will get rid of my back pain.

Fact: The key is doing the *right* workouts that will preserve your back instead of destroying it. I see patients often perplexed by the fact that they take care of their bodies when an "unfit Joe" they know seems to get by with no back trouble at all. The truth is that someone hitting the gym every day without using spine sparing techniques during their workout, will develop cumulative trauma in their discs. Repeatedly bending your back at the gym, followed by long periods of sitting at work, chased down with poorly executed daily tasks such as getting dressed or gardening conspire together to cause the delamination of some of your disc fibers. "Unfit Joe," who sits all day, doesn't experience the same strain on his back that a gym superstar does by aggravating their disc injuries every time they sit. In terms of pain, their spines are better off! The key is not to stop working out! The secret is in changing your default movement patterns so that you can enjoy the benefits of fitness without compromising your back.

Myth: Yoga and Pilates are great ways to alleviate back pain.

Truth: While many doctors and therapists will suggest this type of exercise to their patients because of its "therapeutic" properties, our studies have not supported these claims and in fact have indicated the opposite. While some poses and movements may be beneficial or feel good at the time, there are components of both exercise systems that will aggravate an individual with back conditions. There is no such thing as an exercise program that is beneficial to all back pain sufferers and to broadly prescribe either yoga or pilates to a patient with undefined back pain is, in my opinion, *irresponsible*. Every single exercise should be justified and then modified if necessary to suit each person.

One of my major issues with Pilates is that one of its key principles is to flatten the spine and "imprint" the lower back to the floor when lying down. This deliberate effort to disrupt the spine from its neutral position and "straighten" one of its natural curves is not healthy and blatantly simulates many individuals' mechanism of injury. Some people experience a false sense of relief while going through this motion because it stimulates the back's stretch receptors. In reality this relief is fleeting and pain symptoms typically return with a vengeance due to the stresses placed on your discs.

Another staple of the Pilates regimen is called the "Rollup." This movement is essentially a sit-up that involves segmentally rolling through each joint of the spine. Our science has justified avoiding sit-ups as part of a routine for a healthy spine and the Rollup essentially takes a bad exercise and makes it worse. The exaggerated fashion of this exercise puts an emphasis on moving through the spine, putting unnecessary load and strain on the discs. The real goal should be to minimize spinal movement and instead use our hips as primary centers for motion. This philosophy will allow the back pain to settle.

As we've already discussed, a therapeutic exercise must be recommended that correlates with the results of a detailed assessment. Many doctors mindlessly suggest Pilates, buying into the unexamined orthodoxy that says Pilates is good for the back. This needs to stop. Don't get me wrong. There are many Pilates and Yoga instructors I have met taking my clinical courses and have expertise in matching specific exercises to specific people. These instructors are well aware of the importance of avoiding certain pain triggers and adjusting exercises to prevent the worsening of pain. The bottom line is that if the specific components of Yoga and Pilates are selected and modified for the person doing them, they can help a back patient, but neither of these programs should ever be recommended as a "blanket cure" to all back pain sufferers.

Patient Files: A Yoga master came to my office for a consult. I asked her to show me what made her pain worse. She sat on the floor in a pose, fully twisting her spine, staying there for several minutes. It took her another few minutes to work through the pain to stand up. I stated, "I think I know what is causing your pain – doing that exercise". She was in disbelief. She thought all she needed was to keep forcing more mobility. Then she broke down. She admitted that the traditional practice of Yoga was to remove tension from the body to facilitate transcending of the mind. I pointed out her large boned physique caused much higher spine stress than a thinner-boned person. A thick tree branch shatters much sooner than a thin branch given an equal amount of bend or twist. I think she came to me expecting me to validate her Yoga practice. The only chance she had to become healthy was to stop stressing her painful, sensitized joints to end range. Her way of life and livelihood had just been challenged. Emotionally, this was extremely difficult for her to come to terms with.

Myth: Stretching is good for reducing back pain.

Fact: Although stretching is considered universally beneficial for back pain sufferers, this is an old-fashioned notion that needs challenging.

There is no such thing as a stretch that is good for all patients, just as there is no such thing as a single source of pain. Each back pain case is different, and as such each stretch must be chosen very, very carefully and tailored to the individual. Too often, therapists prescribe stretches that are totally wrong for a patient often with the ultimate goal of improving mobility in the spine. For most back pain sufferers, this is the *opposite* of what they should be doing in order to gain control of their backs.

Physiologically, pulling your knees to your chest, or other similar stretches, triggers the "stretch reflex." This is a neurological phenomenon that reduces pain sensitivity. This provides about 15-20 minutes of pain relief for some, making it a short-term fix. The problem is that in putting your spine in this position, you are aggravating your discs and after you've experienced temporary relief, the pain will return, often worse than before. Thus begins a vicious cycle with a misinformed back patient who thinks their only solution to pain is to "stretch it out," not realizing that this in fact is contributing to their pain. The key is to stop the cycle!

Instead of focusing your energy on stretches that bend the spine, turn instead to stabilizing and controlling the spine. Modifying your daily movements to keep your spine in a "neutral" position as much as possible is a good place to start. In following this path to recovery, your discs will experience less strain, your pain will subside and your mobility will return!

Essentially, when dealing with stretches, avoid any motion that involves pulling your knees to your chest. There are, however, certain stretches for other parts of the body that may aid you on your road to being pain free. We will discuss these later.

Myth: My friend was cured using XYZ therapy – he swears by it. It must be good for me.

Fact: As previously mentioned there is no universal cause or cure for back pain. A method that led to success for a friend may or may not be beneficial to you as your condition is likely different. The following chapters will focus on finding your own pain triggers and matching them to the "treatment" and "dosage" that is best for you.

Myth: Stronger muscles will cure my back pain.

Fact: Therapists often begin strength training early in rehabilitation simply because strength is the easiest attribute to increase and requires very little expertise. Or, curiously they have decided to measure strength as a metric for disability – this is driven by a legal process seeking monetary settlements based on strength loss (or sometimes loss of motion). Too many patients remain long-term patients because of their misguided efforts to train their back strength. In many cases, their training approach needs an overhaul. Think of strength in relation to the body like horsepower in relation to a car. If a souped-up 500 horsepower engine is put inside a dinky, broken down car and then raced around town at top speed, it's only a matter of time before the mega-engine rips the frail frame and suspension to pieces. Similarly, a back patient who has developed a disproportionate amount of strength in relation to their current level of *endurance* can only expect further injury. We have measured this time and time again in strong back patients.

Back injuries are a result of putting a spine under load and then breaking healthy movement form. Maintaining proper movement patterns requires endurance. Therefore, we must always place endurance as a higher priority to strength when it comes to rehabilitating a patient with a spine condition. Only once we have increased our endurance for sustaining healthy movement patterns, and in turn our stability and mobility, should we move on to more aggressive strength training.

Insights from the podium: Mitch owned a couple of world records in powerlifting. The idea is to lift as much weight as possible off the floor. Sooner or later body parts under tension will tear, while those in compression will crush. He split a vertebra that looked as if a woodsman had driven a wedge down into it. After failing several rehab attempts involving strengthening the area, he requested an appointment at our clinic. Immediately it was apparent that his carefree attitude for sloppy movement meant he continually "picked the scab". His continued attempts to regain strength through the pain marked his further progressive decline. What he did have in his favour was a highly developed appreciation for professionalism. He spent the next half year under our guidance following a bone callousing program focussed on bone repair and pristine movement patterns to distress his joints. Nothing else. Then he was able to transition to a strength training program, with impeccable movement patterns. Within another year he was highly competitive once again. We have done this enough times to prove it was not luck.

Myth: Work Hardening Programs help all back pain sufferers get back to work.

Fact: Although these programs are popular with compensation boards and insurance companies, the truth is that although they help some individuals, they often hurt others.

Work Hardening Programs are designed to increase pain tolerance to a degree that enables the injured individual to resume work. The major flaw lies in the philosophy that by creating a simulated work environment, whose activities become more demanding each day, you will increase the pain threshold the worker is able to withstand. While some will respond well to this structure and survive to return to work, others will be driven to more tissue breakdown, worsening their condition. These individuals would be better suited to a more progressive recovery program, one that may require more patience but will deliver better long-term results. Yet most Work Hardening protocols are not permitted to make allowances for individualized rates of progress. This flies in the face of the laws of nature and biology. In the published reports of the effectiveness of Work Hardening Programs, a "dropout rate" is typically listed. Those who were unable to complete the program because their condition worsened would fall under this category and be labelled as "non-compliant" insinuating it was the patient's fault. The truth is that they were given loads beyond their current capacity and their backs were broken down further. These "drop out" cases are typically not included when determining the overall success rate and therefore skew the numbers so they no longer reflect the actual "success rate." Such reports are just fine with the firms and insurance companies as this gives them an excuse to label anyone not suited to the program as "non compliant" and typically leads to the patient being removed from the insurance company's liability list. For many patients this isn't right or just.

Myth: Having a powerful back is protective.

Fact: Power is the product of velocity and force. Essentially power is moving or bending the spine with forceful exertion. Generating power in the spine is highly problematic as it increases the risk of injury. Let's break it down. If spine movement or bending occur at a high velocity, the forces (or *load*) on it must be low in order to avoid injury. Alternatively, if the force being placed on the spine is high, then the velocity must be kept at a low level in order to maintain a low risk of injury. Essentially it is the combined *power*, or levels of velocity in *relation* to force that determine your degree of risk. Studying only force or only velocity in an isolated context hinders your ability to see the bigger picture of what is really putting your back in danger.

Myth: Body building exercises will help with rehabilitation.
Fact: The principles of body building will actually "pollute" a recovery. Bulking up or "hypertrophying" muscles is not the answer to finding pain free function.

More often than not the clinician or therapist directing the rehabilitative resistance training uses *isolation exercises* that target a single muscle. These are usually performed on an exercise machine. An example of a typical recommendation would be for a patient to employ three sets of 10 repetitions in a wide variety of exercises and to perform this resistance training regimen three times per week. The critical question remains: are these bodybuilding resistance training principles consistent with the principles of enhancing ones control of movement and control of their muscles? The answer is a resounding NO!

Worse yet are the choices of exercises prescribed. Consider this oh-too-typical situation: the back-pained patient is told to perform multiple sets of bench presses. This recommendation not only causes pain, but fails to build pain-free ability. As dictated by the laws of physics, from a standing posture an individual can forward-press half of their body weight. I have seen patients who are superstars when it comes to bench-pressing but struggle when trying to push open a steel door at the entrance of our clinic. A better substitute to bench-pressing would be performing pushups on the floor. In our lab, we have measured the mechanics and effectiveness of a plethora of exercises and because of that have been able to determine which will help to rebuild a back, and contrarily which will tear down a back. You will learn which exercises are best suited to your individual case in the upcoming sections of the book.

Myth: I read a study on back pain that stated "Nothing works, just get on with it."
Fact: No single study will reveal the universal solution to a problem as complex as back pain. Controlled trials that attempt to determine a one-size-fits-all cure only work for conditions that are more homogeneous – like diabetes. Because back pain varies so much in cause and ideal treatment between individuals, these types of studies will remain inconclusive. A study on a single intervention method will show on average, no effect – some patients get better and some get worse. But the fact is some got better. What was different with these individuals? If we identify the variables they have in common, we come up with a set of symptoms that respond positively to a specific type of treatment. In studying the varying causes and effects of back pain, and through seeing patients over the years experience their own successes and failures, we have come up with valuable insights on matching the patient with the cure. It is these insights that are shared throughout the rest of the book.

Myth: Foolproof "fix your back in 7 days" or "be pain free in five easy steps" plans are great rehabilitation options.
Fact: At this point we've established that there is no simple, easy cure that will work for everyone. A damaged and painful back cannot be miraculously fixed in a week. Even in the best case scenario, you may *feel* great after a small amount of therapy but all it takes is one relapse of repeating the pain trigger to set you all the way back again. Your task is to manage the damaged tissues through healthy movement patterns in order to remain pain free as you give them time to heal. By following the recommendations here you will join the vast majority of my patients and the patients of the thousands of clinicians I have taught, who never again had an acute episode of back pain.

In Review

- If your Doctor's primary approach to your recovery lies in pain medication, you need different expertise.
- If all you have been given is a list of exercises from your physiotherapist, you need to find a new approach.
- If all you get is "manipulation" from your chiropractor, and you need repeat visits, you need to find a new approach.
- If you ever have a pain-free movement, you have the capability to expand your repertoire of pain-free movements to become pain-free living. You are curable.

Chapter 2

Back to Basics: Getting to Know Your Back and Causes of Pain

Back to Basics

Getting to Know Your Back and Causes of Pain

One of my biggest grievances when speaking to patients about their previous experience with doctors is that they have received either too broad a diagnosis ("lower back pain, here's some meds") or they've come away with little information other than the knowledge that they have "modic changes at L5 or spinal stenosis" or worse, they have degenerative disc disease which does not help direct the cure. In all of these instances the medical "expert" failed to include a crucial component in their assessment of the patient: an explanation of basic injury and pain mechanisms that would guide a solution. Many people come to me with little understanding of how their spine functions, what its role is in relation to the rest of the body, and what all of this means for their individual pain causes. In many cases, this poor practice may be a result of the pressure on doctors to see upwards of forty patients a day, allotting less than ten minutes to each one, forcing them to abbreviate and condense important assessments and explanations. In other cases I believe it is a genuine lack of information and understanding on the doctors' part. Simply put, they just may not have the knowledge and training in back health necessary to provide you with the care you need and deserve.

The first thing we need to establish, is that the spine is not a freestanding pillar, such as Toronto's CN Tower or similar "observation towers" found in Seattle and Auckland, floating among organs and flesh. Instead, we need to think of it more like a radio tower, those tall metallic structures stabilized by guy-wires that are connected to the ground. The function of these guy-wires is similar to that of the network of muscles and ligaments that surround our spinal columns: they provide strength and support. In the case of our backs, these "anchoring" muscles also facilitate mobility. As with any part of our mobile bodies, from our elbows to our jaws, it is not our bones that create motion, but the muscles attached to them. More on these muscles later.

The Neutral Spine

To best understand the actual skeletal structure of the spine, which travels from the base of the skull all the way down to the pelvis, we must look at it in its natural position or "neutral." This position is essentially the spine's "home-base," in which it is in its least stressed position. When in the neutral position the spine is most resilient to the imposed stresses of daily life.

When a healthy spine is in neutral, three natural curves are present:

1. The neck, or ***cervical spine***, which begins in a cavity in the back of the skull and ends approximately where the neck meets the beginning of the torso, curves gently inward toward the front of the body (the medical term for this curve is ***lordosis***).

2. The mid back, or ***thoracic spine***, which begins at the point of the back that intersects the imaginary line connecting the top of your shoulders and extends to the bottom of the ribcage, curves outward away from the lungs (the medical term for this curve is ***kyphosis***).

3. The low back, or ***lumbar spine***, which begins at the base of the ribcage and extends through to the base of the pelvis, or tailbone, curves inward towards the abdominal organs (this curve is also referred to as ***lordosis***).

The spine has 3 sections: the neck or cervical spine; the middle section with the rib cage or thoracic spine; and the low back or lumbar spine. When we think of "sitting up straight" or "standing up straight", there may be the tendency to imagine the spinal column lengthening into a perfectly aligned vertical tower down our backs, but when we feel as though we're "up straight" we're actually "up neutral." This means that good posture, actually involves the presence of each of these three natural curves in the back. The cervical, thoracic and lumbar curves are:

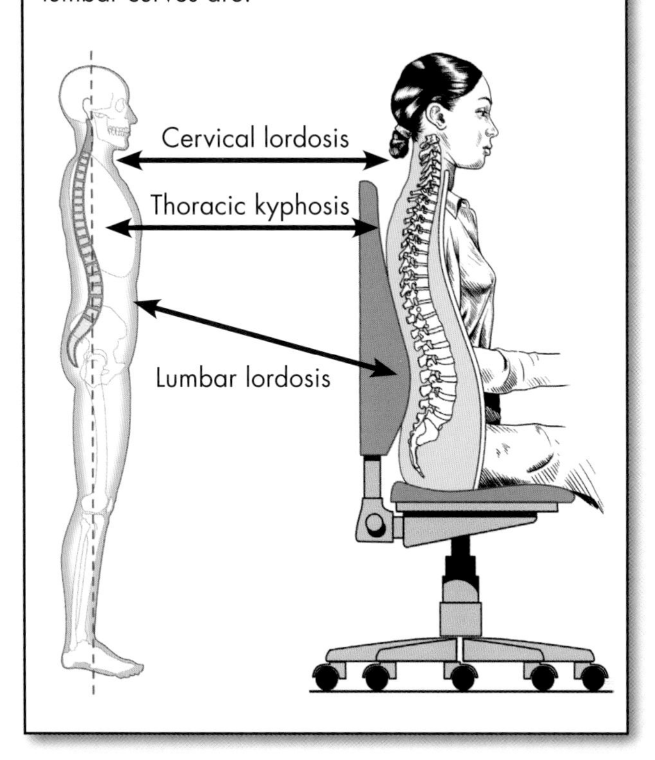

Although motion through the back is only natural and promotes healthy tissue, our spine is at its strongest, most resilient and most supported position when it is in neutral. We will continue to refer back to this position throughout the book.

Bones and Joints (Vertebrae and Discs)

The spinal column is comprised of individual bones called ***vertebra*** that are stacked one on top of the other. The structure of each vertebra includes bony protrusions called ***processes*** that serve as anchoring points for important muscles and ligaments. If you run your finger down your back, the small bumps you feel are actually these processes. The actual bodies of the vertebrae sit several inches inward. Between the vertebrae are the ***discs***, which are not bones but more like "bone spacers." Each disc has tough outer rings of collagen, the same material that forms the body's ligaments and tendons. Inside these hoops of collagen, each disc contains a gel called the ***nucleus***. Within its collagen "pocket" each nucleus is pressurized, which gives it the ability to bend – think of a car tire who's internal air pressure allows it to support the weight of the car. The actual joints of the spine are found behind the discs, on the side of the spine farthest away from the organs. These are called the ***facet joints***, of which there are two for every disc. The facet joints guide the motion of each vertebra as the spine bends, twists and turns, supporting the ***shear*** forces. Like other joints in the body, they glide over one another to facilitate smooth movement patterns.

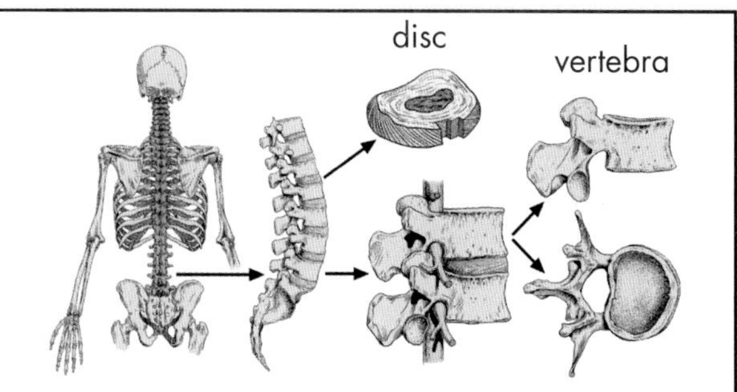

The lumbar spine is in the low back, comprised of bony vertebrae with discs that provide the ability to move. The body's main nerve pathway travels in a canal down the middle of the spine with roots that outlet at each joint. These are what get irritated or pinched with injury and overuse. The vertebrae have bony prominences called processes that allow muscles and ligaments to attach with better leverage to create both movement and stability for the spinal column.

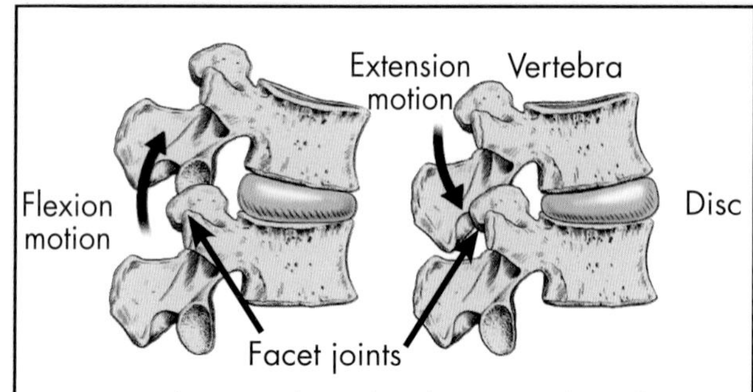

Two vertebrae with a disc between them form a motion unit, so that there are many that make up the full spine. The disc has a pressurized gel-like nucleus that carries the loads down the spine while allowing bending motion. There are two additional joints to each motion unit called the facet joints that guide spine movements. If overused with too many repeated bends and twists they become irritated and painful, and eventually arthritic. Further, if the disc becomes damaged, the facet joints will wear out faster.

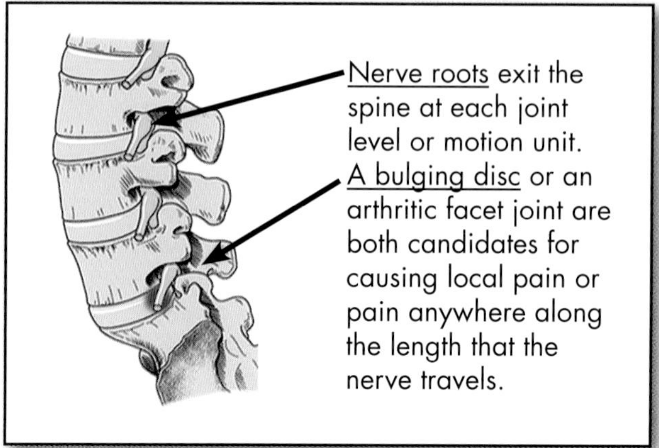

Nerve roots exit the spine at each joint level or motion unit. A bulging disc or an arthritic facet joint are both candidates for causing local pain or pain anywhere along the length that the nerve travels.

If you bend the spine too far and too often the spines discs will eventually crack (or delaminate) and eventually they will break. Paradoxically larger spines crack sooner as the bending stresses are higher (you can bend a thin willow branch much more than a thick branch). This is why people with a thicker spine get back damage faster performing situps, when a slightly built person will survive much longer – exercises affect different body types very differently!

Nerves

The spine houses the main spinal cord which runs from the brain, down the spine, with roots exiting at each spinal level. These sense pain and control movement and control function of your various organs. Damage to the spine irritates or pinches the nerve roots causing back pain, as well as causing pain and numbness in distal parts of the body linked with that particular nerve. Disc bulges and arthritic bone are examples of things that can cause not only back pain but buttock, leg and foot pain.

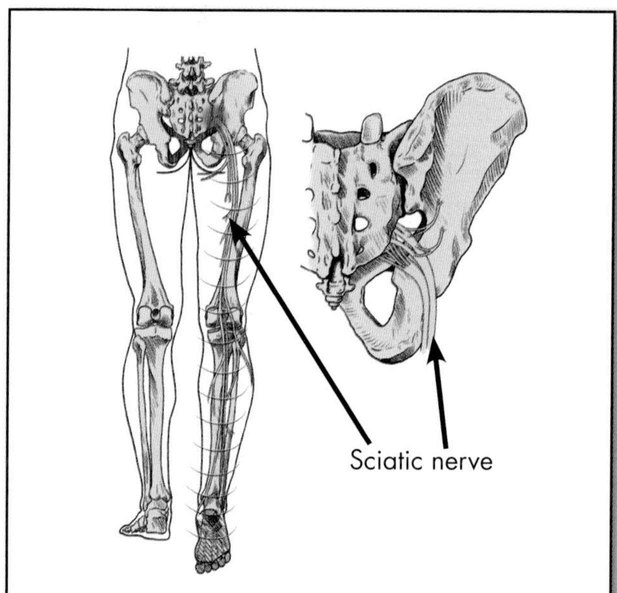

Collections of lumbar nerve roots form major nerves. The sciatic nerve exits from the lower two lumbar levels that when irritated can cause pain in the buttocks behind the hip joint, down the posterior thigh, down the calf, around the ankle and through the foot to the toes. While not shown, nerve roots from the upper three lumbar levels form the femoral nerve that can cause radiating symptoms down the front of the thigh. The point being that all of these symptoms originate from damage and irritation in the lumbar spine.

Nerves are like ropes in that they have small movements along their length as the body moves. If the nerve is pinched, or friction is created along their length, pain often results – the exercise programs described in these pages are scientifically designed to reduce this irritation and common cause of pain.

Nerves get sensitized with mechanical irritation from injury and poor movements. I will guide you to reduce their sensitivity by reducing the irritation.

Muscles

In order to understand how best to deal with pain by choosing better motions, postures and loads we need to understand how muscles actually work. We then need to focus on finding pain-free movements. It is important that we speak the same language. I'll need to share some essential, fundamental anatomy and anatomical terms and phrases here. Some of these may be new to you and some you may have heard before, but using the proper terminology and talking in specifics is a fundamental step in ultimately equipping you with the tools you will need to become your own back mechanic, so please bear with me.

As previously noted, repeated spine bending will eventually lead to delaminations in the layers of the discs. It is important to note that the muscles play a protective role. They are arranged around the spine and designed primarily to stop spinal motion. Torso muscles that are flaccid and weak, or out of balance with one another, allow back problems.

Consider the abdominal wall in front of the torso and its relationship to the spinal column. The rectus abdominis is the frontal abdominal wall muscle and is commonly known as the "six-pack". Anchored to the rectus are the muscles that form the lateral abdominal wall, the obliques. This special arrangement forms "hoops" around the torso, or core. Engineering analysis reveals this very cleverly designed structure acts as a spring: an energy storage and recovery device. This enables you to throw, kick, jump and even walk. It allows the powerful hips to transmit their forces through this spring-loaded core, sparing the spine while enhancing function.

Many pained people do not utilize this principle. As well, too many individuals train this group of muscles as they would their biceps – by taking the muscles through a range of motion. They are making a mistake – a big painful mistake.

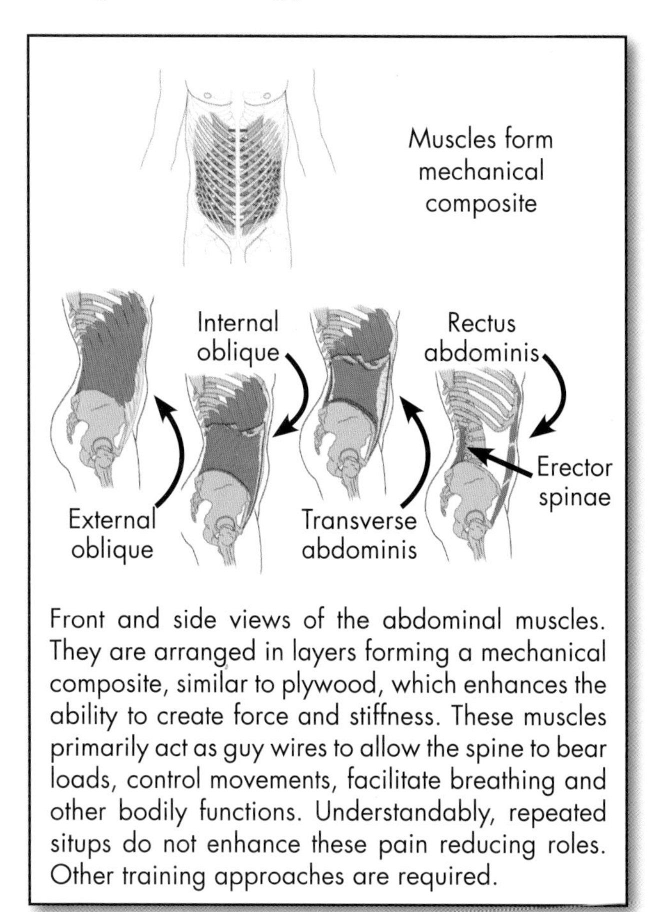

Front and side views of the abdominal muscles. They are arranged in layers forming a mechanical composite, similar to plywood, which enhances the ability to create force and stiffness. These muscles primarily act as guy wires to allow the spine to bear loads, control movements, facilitate breathing and other bodily functions. Understandably, repeated situps do not enhance these pain reducing roles. Other training approaches are required.

The muscles of the back include the spinal erectors (including multifidus, longissimus, iliocostalis), quadratus lumborum, latisimus dorsi, rhomboids, trapezius, and many smaller ones close to the spine itself. The erectors stiffen and support the tendency to bend forward. They perform this function while also balancing some of the ***shear*** forces. But in order to do this the spine must be in its un-bent, or neutral posture. Latissimus is a very important muscle for stabilizing the spine to make it more resilient while enhancing performance. It is part of the family of muscles involved in lifting, pulling and carrying tasks.

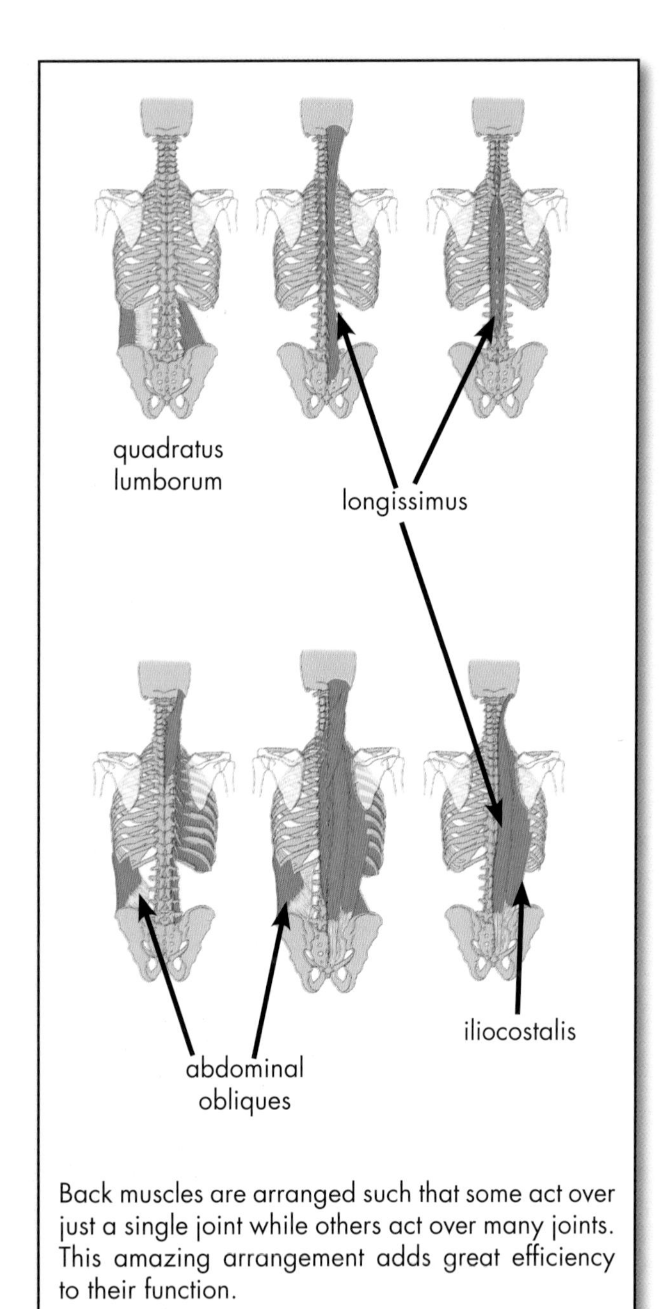

Back muscles are arranged such that some act over just a single joint while others act over many joints. This amazing arrangement adds great efficiency to their function.

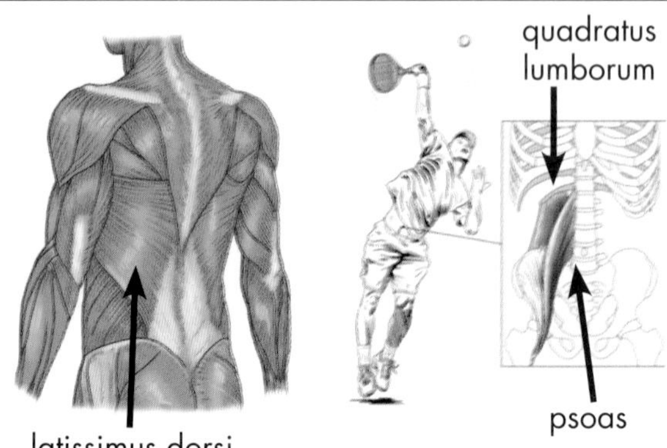

The back muscles work together enhancing one another so that the whole system is stronger and stiffer than the sum of the parts. The posterior guy wire system helps to stop motion in some situations, and create movement in others. It also supports shear loads to ensure safe handling of loads.

The quadratus lumborum forms the lateral guy wires allowing activities such as walking, and sporting moves. The psoas allows the hip to flex without damaging the spine.

The spine is linked to the legs via the pelvis. The important muscles here are the psoas, iliacus, and the muscles that span the hip such as the gluteal muscles, quadriceps and hamstrings. These muscles are both unique and inseparable. While they influence the spine and move the leg about the hip joint, they respond differently to back and hip pain. For example, pain often inhibits the gluteal muscles during hip extension causing the hamstring muscles to pick up the difference. This has several harmful consequences for both the back and hip joints. Specifically, when the hamstring muscles become dominant, they push the head of the femur (leg bone) into the front of the hip joint leading to pain during a deep squat. This example explains why symptoms often form patterns. It also explains why comprehensive rehabilitation for the back involves not only back muscles but also those for the hips, shoulders, legs and arms.

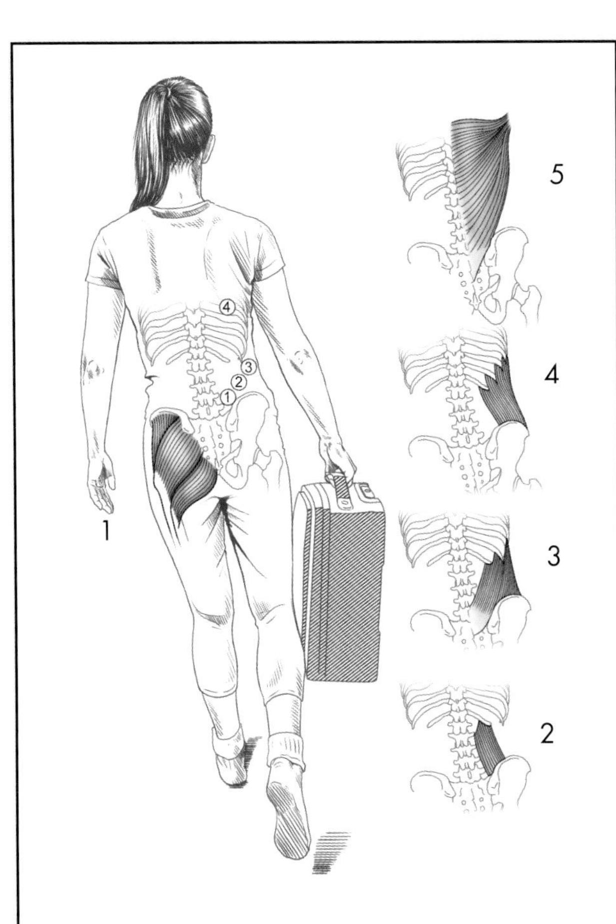

Carrying is a good task to illustrate the role of many muscles. The gluteal muscles of the hip help support the pelvis to allow leg swing – they also extend the hip. On the other side of the body the quadratus lumborum (2) assists this role of holding up the pelvis. The internal oblique (3) muscle stops the pelvis from tilting and arrests twist motion in the torso to allow the hip to power leg swing. The external oblique (4) performs the same role only in the other twist direction. The latissimus dorsi (5) links the shoulder to the spine creating stiffness to control bending.

Poor functioning of any of these muscles will compromise the back and eventually result in pain.

No muscle performs just a single function. Thus, the notion of a muscle being a "spine extensor" misguides rehabilitation. First and foremost the flexible spinal column must be stiffened to allow it to bear load. The muscles work together in various patterns to ensure this vital "sufficient stability". Only then can the muscles be coordinated to create motion, and support loads. Muscles often span several joints meaning that their action at one joint is constrained by its role at another. One cannot simply try to change one muscle without affecting the entire muscular "orchestra". By the same token the orchestra must play with all players in tune with each member, at the correct volume and at the correct tempo and time. Muscle function follows the same rules.

On one hand it is all very complicated and just short of magical. But on the other, there are easily identifiable features of perturbed function associated with pain that we can correct with quite simple exercises that will "re-educate" pain-free patterns. Herein lies the problem with body building exercises for back pain. They fail to create movement competency in patterns that produce pain-free function. The exercises here have been proven to create movement competency and a balance to ensure pain-free function.

Connective Tissues

Ligaments, joint capsules and fascia comprise the connective tissues. They function to limit end-range motion and in the case of the fascia, hold the parts together. But they do so much more. These tissues can become painful when they are strained with the joints at the end-range of motion. This happens with repetitive motion and activity. The pain can be local but in some cases cause distal symptoms. Characteristically, this pain generally has a slow onset and lingers on. It does not have a stabbing onset, nor a quick recovery, which is more characteristic of a disc bulge.

The fascia is made of tough sheets that look like multiple layers of food wrap and cover muscles and bundles of muscles. It can create a "swirly" pain around the shoulders, low back and hip area. Interestingly, syndromes such as fibromyalgia where the fascia is highly sensitized, can result from trauma that re-wires the brains' sensitivity and triggering to pain. The best results we have had with these patients resulted from working with the patient on whatever movements they can perform pain-free, and then slowly and patiently expanding the pain-free repertoire. Basically, the approach is to teach the brain pain-free movement and overwrite the painful pathways.

Patient Files: Dania came to her appointment having recently been released from prison. She witnessed her husband being murdered while she was traumatized during a crime. She had back pain but reported the "swirly" symptoms consistent with fibromyalgia. She was dismissed as a faker, a psychological case. Yet physical and emotional trauma is so commonly associated with fibromyalgia. I led her outside of my office to observe her walking gait in the hallway. Her gait exuded the demeanor of someone who was downtrodden – her shoulders slumped and she had chronically contracted back muscles causing cramping pain. Then a student came around the corner startling her. The striations of muscle contraction jumped out of her shoulders revealed with her tank top. She collapsed with a searing headache and back pain.

Slowly we taught her simple pain-free movements and corrected her posture. We "taught" her neural system to tolerate more movement without pain. While not completely cured after several months she was able to become resilient, then was able to add exercise. She regained her swagger. But it was understanding the cause of her unique symptoms that pointed the therapeutic approach in the right direction. Her doctors missed all of these critical variables, lacked understanding of the cause, and worse yet, they blamed her for their inability to help her.

Movement and Load

This is where all of the basic anatomy comes together and we understand how the back works as an entire unit. It is this section where the concept of load is introduced and explained. Concepts of stiffness vs. mobility, and how different movement patterns cause pain are addressed.

What is load?

When we pick up an object, or push on a heavy door, forces are applied to the body. These are direct loads on the body. But even more important are the internal loads. Consider holding 5 pounds (2.2 kilos) in your hand. The elbow flexor muscles support the object in this posture by contracting. But they have a line of action much closer to the joint (about 1/15th) meaning that their force is 15 times the weight of the object, in this case 75 pounds (34 kilos). The flexor muscles span the joint so 75 pounds (34 kilos) squeezes the joint. In this way the elbow joint sustains 75 pounds (34 kilos) of load just to enable 5 pounds (2.2 kilos) to be held in the hands.

Holding a 50-pound (23 kilo) object would cause 750 pounds (340 kilos) of force on the elbow bones (close to half a ton)! The spine experiences the same type of load magnification. Bending over to pick up an object in your hands requires your back muscles to contract. Since they are close to the spine they contract with great force which is imposed on the spine joints. To bend forward with just body weight results in about 1/3rd of a ton of force! This is why it is so important to use joint sparing mechanics – keep objects being lifted close to the body, be aware of repeated and sustained postures that result in these excessive spine loadings. (More on this in a couple of chapters.)

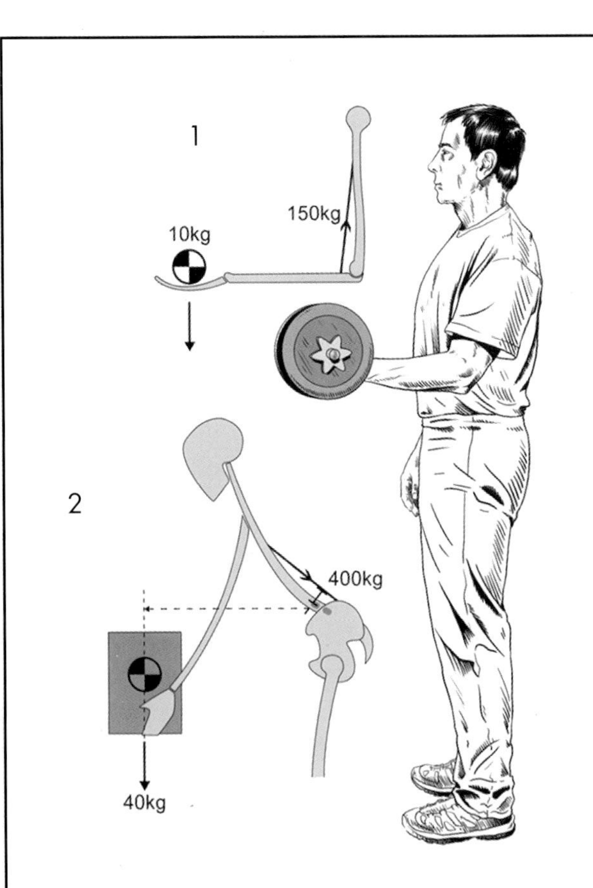

Holding 10 kg in the hand requires the elbow flexors to create 150 kg of force because of their mechanical disadvantage (1). These muscles span the joint imposing this large force on the elbow. In the same way the back muscles impose their forces on the spine (2). The further away the object held in the hands is from the spine, the higher the back muscle forces, the higher the crushing load on the spine. It is not uncommon for the spine to experience half a ton of compressive load when objects are lifted some distance from the body – even surprisingly light objects. This highlights the importance of proper movement mechanics.

How posture determines spine load and pain

Your postures and movements determine the loads, and stress, on your joints. This stress influences your pain. Understanding the cause of compression and shear force, together with bending, will guide you in making the choices necessary to avoid pain.

Compression forces squeeze the joints. Compression is largely the result of muscle force. This is why the choice of posture and movement and the choice of exercise are so important.

Shear forces are perpendicular to compression forces. They cause joints to rub across one another. This is unstable motion. Shear forces develop from certain applied loads and postures but are lessened by muscle anatomy and the choice of spine posture.

When bending over, shear force is increased to the spine. Those with shear induced pain will do better to avoid this. Those with sensitivity to compression will also be advised to avoid forward bending as this creates more muscle force which is transferred to the spine along the compressive axis.

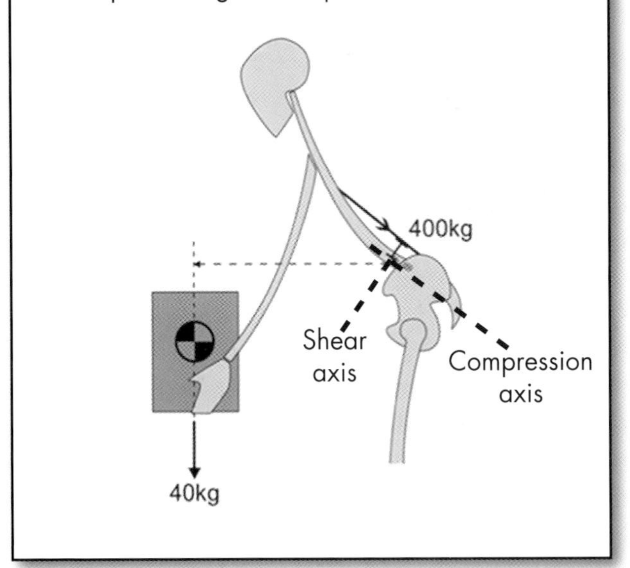

Bending

The spine bends much like a bending rod. The discs deform to allow the bending motion. Imagine taking a wire coat hanger and bending it back and forth over and over. Eventually the metal will fatigue and break. The spine experiences the same cumulative effect with repeated bending. Eventually the disc fibers will crack and the inner gel-like nucleus will seep through the outer wall. This is the source of pain in many people, particularly those who are under the age of 55. The key to avoiding this type of pain is to bend about the hips rather than the spine. ***The hips are designed to bend (ball and socket joints) while the spine is a flexible rod that becomes painful with repeated bending.***

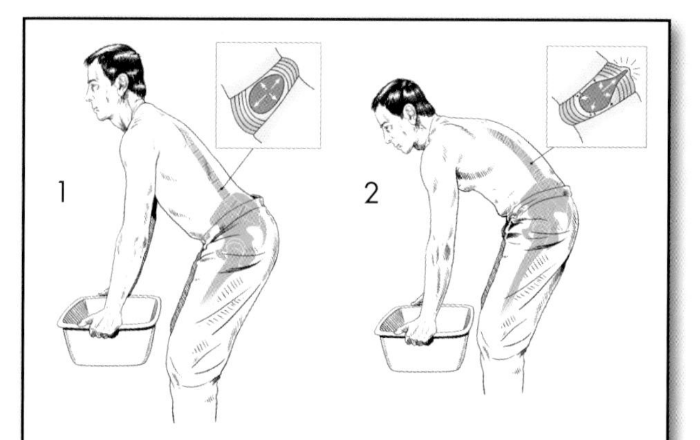

In both pictures the person is doing the same task of holding a tub, but their risk of back injury is substantially different. (1) Notice he has flexed, or bent, using his hips – his spine did not bend or change shape. The natural wedge shape of his lumbar disc did not change so there is no additional stress, or risk. (2) Notice, in contrast to the left panel, he elected to bend his spine together with some hip bending. His spinal disc is bent creating large posterior stresses. Over time the nucleus of the disc will travel through the layers of the disc annulus as they separate under the repeated stresses. This is what causes a disc bulge. **The avoidance strategy is to bend at the hips!**

Muscles of the torso and back are fundamentally different than limb muscles

These complex muscle patterns are controlled by the body's computer – our brain is in charge. But the control of the torso muscles is fundamentally different than the control of muscles of the limbs because limb muscles create motion while torso muscles primarily stop motion.

Consider the simple act of walking where leg movement would not be possible without stiffness and stability to stop motion in the spine. This "fixes" the pelvis to lift one leg and swing it forward while supporting the bodyweight on the other leg. Without a spine muscle named the quadratus lumborum (a muscle each side of the lumbar spine) to assist in stiffening the torso and pelvis, the leg could not be swung and walking would be extremely difficult. The quadratus neither shortens nor lengthens, rather it activates simply to stiffen and stop motion. This is why we will train this muscle, essential for spine health, with no motion using the unique exercises found in this book.

Patient Files: Dennis played rugby and "messed up" his back only when running at speed and changing direction. Assessment revealed his side bridge exercise score was much less than the front plank and birddog score – revealing a lateral endurance deficit to his core musculature. His quadratus lumborum muscle was not trained to the level of the rest of his core musculature. Performing "suitcase carry" exercises trained this muscle without changing its length, perfectly addressing his pain trigger. Dennis regained his ability to play his sport with passion. I will show you these details.

Let's also consider the mechanics associated with opening a door: the hips and legs create a root into the ground as the arm reaches forward and pulls on the door handle. These upper and lower body forces work to twist the spine. But the torso muscles stiffen against the twisting tendency to prevent this motion. This is known as a "spine-sparing" movement strategy.

Thus limb movement from limb muscles requires a stiffened torso. This principle is at the root of great athletic performance.

Those who allow the spine to bend instead of taking advantage of the motion and power production in the hips will either hurt their backs or limit their performance. During daily activity the same rule applies. If the torso muscles are not stiffened and engaged when you perform a simple act, like reaching for a door handle to open a door, the spine would be forced to bend causing stress and eventual pain.

The implications are great. We train the core to stop motion and train the shoulders and hips to create motion. This requires two entirely different philosophies and approaches. Many experts mistakenly train these two diametrically opposed functions in the same fashion. This can cause pain, poor performance and even injury. Optimally the spine and torso need to move in a coordinated ballet; we seek to optimize the linkage between the high motion joints and the arm and leg segments.

The body needs to be kept in balance: weak links need to be addressed. All the bodily component parts (including the spine) need to work together in a functional, pain-free fashion. Remember that the core is different – it needs to be trained differently from other distal parts of the body because limb muscles create motion while torso muscles primarily stop motion.

Muscle force and stiffness

Some may misunderstand spine muscle flexibility as being the key to health when it is really "stiffness". This is akin to firmness. The firmness you would develop if you were expecting a punch to the midsection.

When muscles contract they create force and also stiffness. Sometimes the muscles are activated to add force and other times it is to create stiffness. All limb movement needs a stiffened core. The stiffness allows your spine to support loads. Imagine a stack of oranges. Placing a weight on top would cause the stack to crumble and fall. But if toothpicks were stuck into the oranges and strings connected from the toothpicks down to the ground, the stack will be stiffened and not crumble. The spine works this way, complete with the bony posts on the vertebrae that attach to the muscles. This essential stiffness is what the core muscles provide.

Many who prescribe exercise fail to recognize these unique features of back muscle function. Isolating and exercising the lower back muscles while performing therapeutic, back isolation, progressive resistance exercises actually amplifies back pain. To reduce pain, rotational torso motion must originate from the hips and shoulders and not come about through rotation and flexion of the spinal column.

Thus, the definition of "core" muscles includes all that attach the pelvis, spine, and ribcage. But we must also add those muscles that cross the hips.

The practical implications from this are profound: *therapeutic exercises for the spine and core muscles follow different rules than those for the hips and limbs. The core needs special attention because the core is different.*

- The muscles of the limbs (and hips) are designed to create motion.
- The muscles of the core are (primarily) designed to stop motion.
- The torso muscles follow a different set of rules from limb muscles.

Spine stability versus mobility

We have seen that stiffness is necessary to prevent buckling collapse of the spinal column when supporting a load. We have also seen how a stiffened torso facilitates limb movement. This essential stiffness also acts as a corset around the spinal joints to stop micro-movements that cause pain. A stiffened spine is a stable and functional one.

Stability comes from muscle stiffness. The way the muscles contract all around the spine determines stability – not strength. Injury causes laxity in the joints, and pain. Insufficient stiffness allows micro-movements that cause pain. It is critical, that we create an effective muscular "guy-wire system", and girdle, all around the spine.

Stiffness, and muscular effort need to be "tuned to the task" – if we expend too much effort, we add crushing loads to the spine.

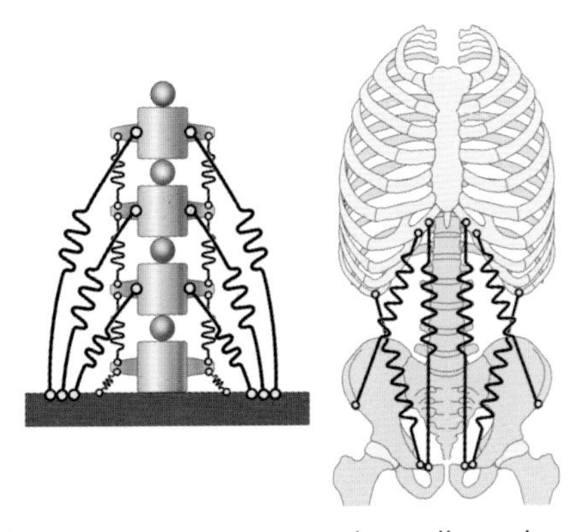

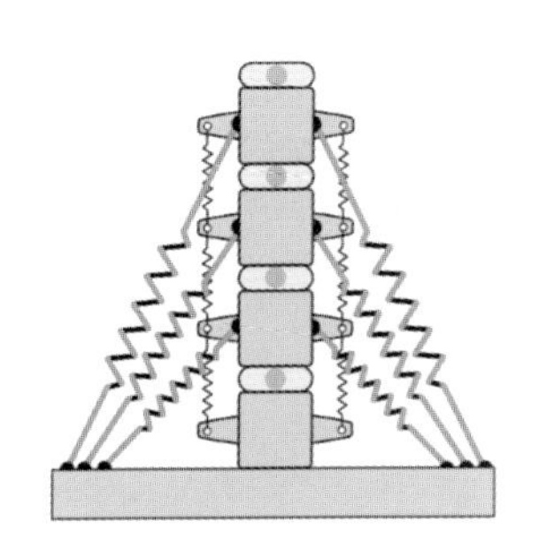

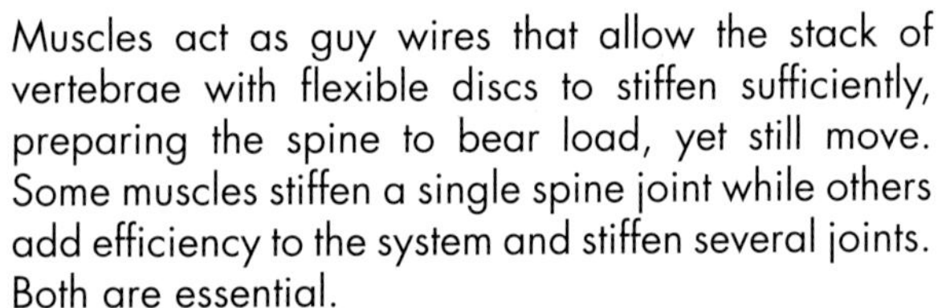

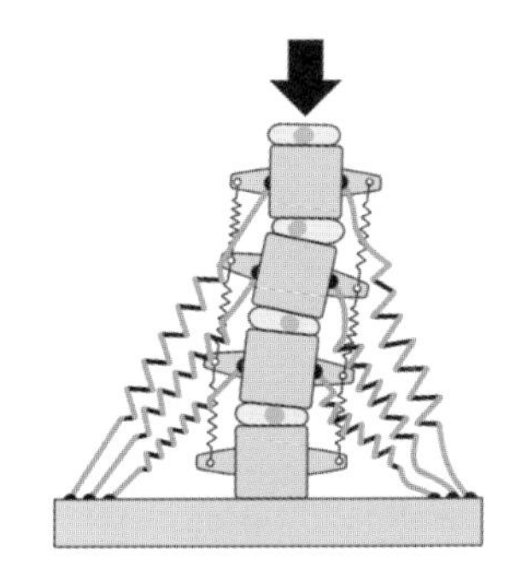

Muscles act as guy wires that allow the stack of vertebrae with flexible discs to stiffen sufficiently, preparing the spine to bear load, yet still move. Some muscles stiffen a single spine joint while others add efficiency to the system and stiffen several joints. Both are essential.

Insufficient stiffness can allow the spine to buckle, causing pain. In contrast, too much stiffness only crushes the spine. Stiffness must be "tuned" akin to a dimmer switch on a light – not an On/Off switch. I will show you how to "tune" your muscles to do this pain-free.

Yet with enough effort (and muscle tension) we ensure stiffness sufficient to prevent joint micro-movement and the resulting pain. The right exercises done at the right time in the right way will train spinal control and stability.

Achieving sufficient stability throughout the day requires muscle activity for longer, not shorter, periods of time. The contraction levels are not substantial, but they are often sustained. This is why stability training begins with endurance training. There exists a widespread misconception amongst clinicians that strength comes before endurance but this is backwards: **endurance needs to be acquired first, strength second. Too much strength too soon creates problems for back-pained individuals.**

Still, many believe that the key to alleviating their pain is to enhance the mobility in their spine, while the opposite is most often true. Isn't it ironic that some doctors give blanket recommendations such as to go swimming, or do yoga or Pilates? While some patients will benefit from some yoga and Pilates exercises, only an assessment of their pain triggers will reveal which ones, if any. Mobility is necessary at the shoulders and hips. Most back pain is best addressed by stiffening, not mobilizing the spine when performing tasks that impose spine load.

Too many people suffer needlessly because they have been given the wrong simple activity instruction.

What activity advice have you received?

Understanding Injury Mechanisms

Pain sensitivity is a direct result of overloading the various anatomical parts of the spine with inappropriate movement. There is a definite cause and effect relationship. Recognizing and avoiding the various injury mechanisms is essential to living a pain-free life. In certain cases there is also a genetic component that makes someone more susceptible to certain back conditions. For example, the North American Inuit experience higher fracture rates because of their genetically thin "pars bones," and there are more reported cases of pars fractures or spondylolisthesis in their community because of their genetic predisposition. This being said, all back pain can be managed. By understanding your pain trigger you can begin to understand the key to its abolishment or even avoid developing an injury to begin with. This is our ultimate goal.

Let's take a look at some of the most common back injuries, their causes and some tips on how to avoid them.

Disc Bulges (a.k.a. Herniation, Sequestration, Slipped Disc): This injury occurs when a disc in between two vertebrae develops a bulge which then presses on a nerve. There are two pain onset patterns: one is a slow onset associated with chronic spine flexion patterns such as when sitting; while the other is a sharp "stabbing" onset associated with a forward bend such as picking up a pencil from the floor. An acute crisis usually lasts about 2 weeks. The bulge triggers an inflammatory process that will resolve but unbeknownst to you, you caused it! Learning to avoid the cause is the key. A disc bulge will fit into one of three basic categories.

The first and most common is a focused bulge somewhere around the periphery of the disc. This is caused by repeatedly bending the spine in the direction away from the bulge. For example, a bulge on the posterior left side of the disc indicates that the spine was repeatedly bent forward and to the right. This type of disc bulge is often found in those holding occupations that involve repeated movements (such as loading and unloading a truck or digging with a shovel) as well as in athletes and sometimes in individuals with asymmetric hips (meaning one is stiffer than the other) causing the person to move in a dominant direction.

With this particular type of disc bulge, there is a number of tolerable, or safe bends possible before pain or injury strikes. This number of bends is reduced when movement is performed with more load. The good news is that you have the power to reduce the bulge. An example of healthy movement would be the cat-camel exercise, which involves moving the spine from a rounded, to arched posture while on all fours on the ground. The disc bulge will remain unharmed because there is very little amount of compressive load involved in this exercise. Contrarily, when standing and bending the spine forward to pick something off the floor, high spine compression is caused by the large extensor muscles that are activated. You can eliminate this risk by bending around the hips rather than the spine. You can see how this type of bulge is "dynamic", meaning that your choice of movement pattern will decrease the bulge, or increase it worsening the pain. This is the good news – you can actually control this type of bulge and get it to shrink back down to size.

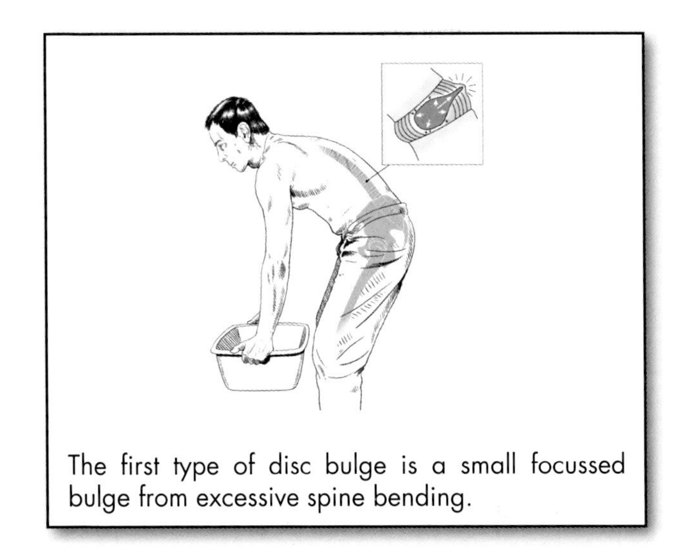

The first type of disc bulge is a small focussed bulge from excessive spine bending.

The second type of disc bulge is a result of a disc losing height. Like a tire that has let some air escape, the flattened disc bulges on all sides. These bulges are more difficult to shrink. Approaches to reducing pain are different for this type. The key for success is to identify the pain-causing activity and eliminate it, then build pain-free movement patterns and turn them into habits instead.

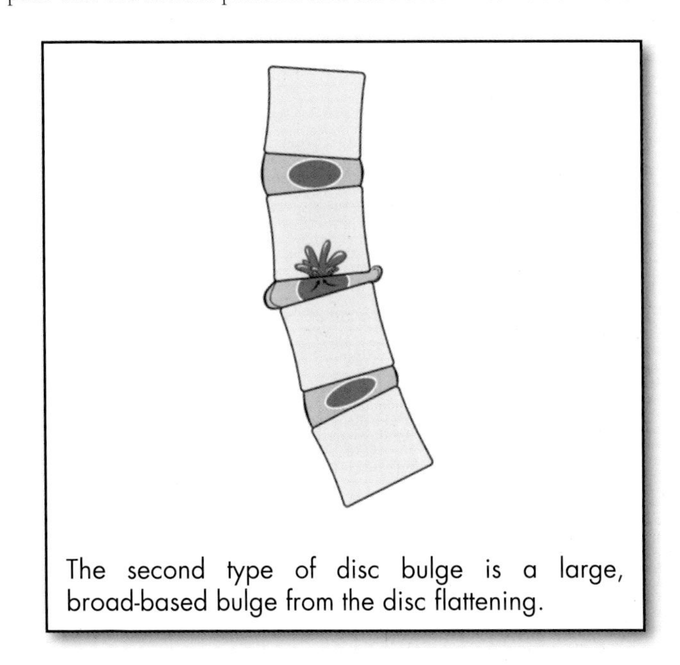

The second type of disc bulge is a large, broad-based bulge from the disc flattening.

The third type of disc bulge is actually a disc tear. The outer disc is made of concentric rings of collagen similar to the layers of an onion. These layers can separate and the nucleus gel from the middle of the disc works its way into the opening fissure between the layers. This type of disc bulge is usually a result of excessive twisting through the spine. The solution? Avoid twisting! The majority of people don't realize how many times throughout the day they unconsciously twist. Making a conscious effort to avoid twisting during activities such as unloading groceries from the car, will alleviate most of the symptoms associated with this type of bulge. Over time the tissue will gristle and not cause pain.

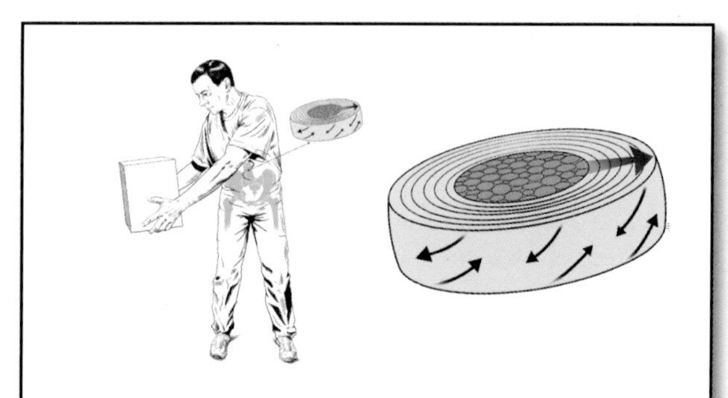

The third type of disc damage is caused by repeated twisting stresses. First, bending initiates a weakening in the annulus (the outer rings), then twisting causes the concentric layers to separate. This forms a disc tear. This requires different treatment protocols.

In summary, disc bulges generally change shape as a function of your movement habits. Learning to hinge forward about the hips rather than bending the spine is the key. Through proper exercise, movement and posture, disc bulges can be made less painful – usually pain-free.

End Plate Damage and the Flattened Disc: When the spine is compressed to a point of injury, the first place to experience damage is the bone of the vertebrae. Micro-fractures occur just under the growth plate, which then allows the endplate to crack. Often times, if the crack is large enough, the nucleus gel escapes into the vertebra, causing the disc to flatten. It also instigates a painful inflammatory response inside the vertebra causing central "boring" pain in the back. In this scenario, it is best to avoid activities that place compression on the spine such as lifting weights or bending forward.

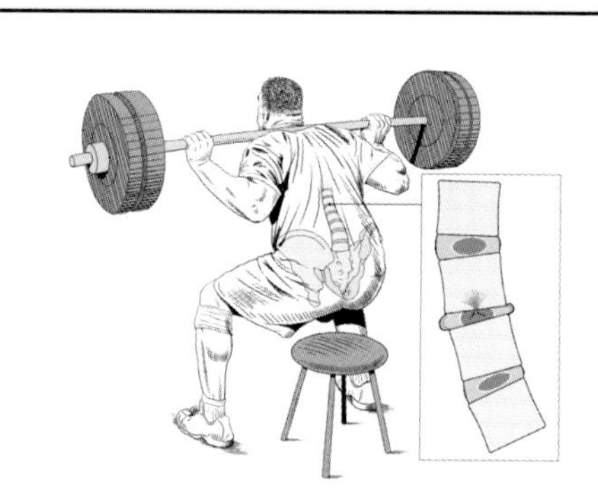

Under excessive compressive loads, the endplates that form the top and bottom of each disc get stressed to the point that they fail. They are no longer able to contain the pressurized nucleus. The crack or split in the endplate allows the pressurized nucleus to escape into the vertebral body. This can cause painful inflammatory responses, a flattened disc, compressed nerve roots. In other words, this injury can instigate a host of pain triggers.

Degenerative Disc Disease: This is a very vague disorder title given to patients who a doctor believes have developed a condition that causes their discs to break down at their own accord. While this is a common diagnosis – it is almost always a misdiagnosis. A radiologist will often make this conclusion upon seeing that a disc has flattened or is losing water content and is thus "drying out." Loss of water content in the disc occurs naturally with aging, it is not a disease. If the "degenerative disc disease" diagnosis is made due to the appearance of one or two specific discs, this is likely an indication that damage or injury has occurred in one particular area in the spine. In these cases the individual disc injury needs to be addressed directly. True early degeneration occurs at many levels throughout the spine, not just one. The paradox is that in such cases, as the discs lose water content, the spine naturally stiffens and over time the discogenic pain disappears. The good news is that the patient's spine will grow out of pain on its own, the bad news is that the spine becomes a bit stiffer making activities like putting your socks on in the morning a little more challenging.

Spondylolisthesis: This term indicates a slippage of one vertebra on another. When this happens, it is usually the top vertebra slipping forward on its lower partner (a backwards slip is known as a retrolisthesis). Usually a bone in the neural arch, behind the vertebrae, is fractured allowing the slip to occur. Pain from a spondylolisthesis typically is continual causing a generally "grumpy" back. Extension movement in particular causes more irritation and can flare the condition into substantial pain. These fractures are the result of excessive bending and twisting through the spine, pushing it to its maximum range. Spondylolisthesis is common among gymnasts, cricket bowlers and some weight training individuals who repeatedly bend their spines while under heavy loads (football linemen are a prime example). Avoiding this mechanism is fairly straight forward – avoid repeated full range of motion of the spine (in other words pushing it to its maximum capacity in flexion or extension), particularly when under load. Sufferers of this condition should avoid activities and postures that place a shear load on the spine (like arching back, kettlebell swings, swimming), as well as things that involve excessive bending motions (like picking things up with a flexed-rounded spine).

Sciatica: Sciatica refers to pain that originates from the spine but is felt along the sciatic nerve into the buttocks and down the back of the leg. The sciatic nerve runs down the back of the thigh, down the shin to the toes, and can be traced back to the nerve roots that exit the spine at the L4/5 and L5/S1 levels. The pain you feel in your buttocks and legs is a product of the sciatic nerve being pinched. In younger patients, the pinch can usually be attributed to a disc bulge (see above section on disc bulges). In an older patient, however, the pinching more likely derives from a bone spur. The key to eliminating sciatic pain depends on the cause of the nerve pinch. Both categories of sciatica can be influenced by posture and spine load. However, the approaches to treatment differ. More on this later.

Femoral nerve pain: Pain felt travelling down the front of the thigh is often from a pinched femoral nerve. Hip joint pain also can travel down the thigh but follows a medial tract (more inner thigh). This particular nerve exits the spine at the upper lumbar spine joints. Patients experiencing this kind of pain should follow the same treatment course as those with sciatic nerve pain, with some minor tuning.

Forward shift

4th

5th

In this example of spondylolisthesis, the 4th lumbar vertebra has shifted forward on the 5th vertebra. This narrows the nerve root opening pinching the nerve, causing both local and radiating pain. All motion becomes painful.

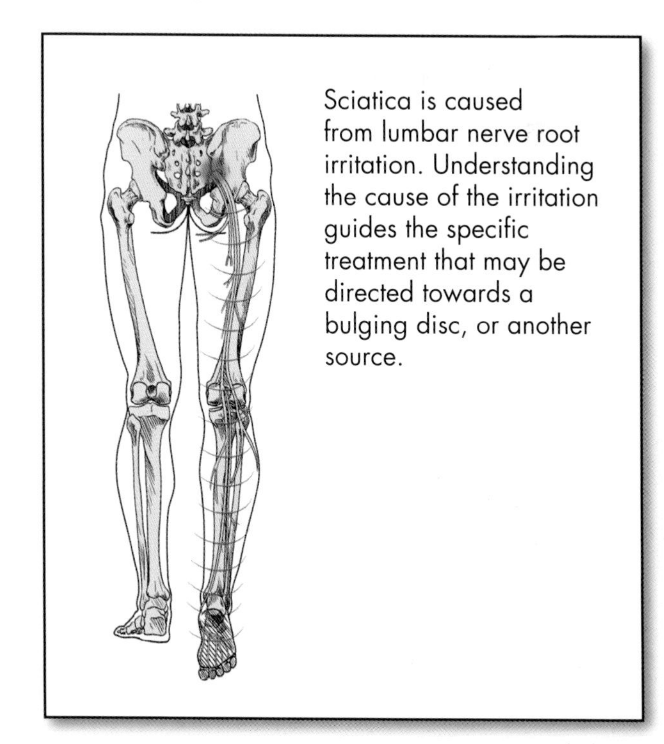

Sciatica is caused from lumbar nerve root irritation. Understanding the cause of the irritation guides the specific treatment that may be directed towards a bulging disc, or another source.

Radiating sensations: These particular perceptions of pain can be felt over the skin (dermatones) and in certain muscles (myotomes). These can usually be traced back to nerve pinches in the lumbar spine. You may notice foot numbness during or following specific activities or after spending time in certain postures. The key to alleviating the pain lies in identifying and avoiding these triggers. Beware that not all sensations have connections to spine issues. A dull ache felt down the middle thigh, through the bone, for example, is an indicator of hip joint pathology. Blood supply compromise (claudication) is another common cause of radiating symptoms. Be sure to check in with a family doctor to rule out these other possible health concerns.

Stenosis: This term refers to a "narrowing" of the canals in the spine where nerves travel. The narrowing can be caused by a number of things, from protruding disc material to arthritic bone to hypertrophied ligaments. Stenosis often results in sciatica and the radiating symptoms noted above. Several coping strategies will be introduced that, in many cases, will eliminate symptoms.

Muscle Pain: Perceived pain in the back muscles is rarely indicative of a muscle "sprain" or a "tear" as many doctors are so quick to declare. The muscle relaxants they would prescribe for this type of pain are nothing but a temporary quick-fix. Although sprains and tears do happen, they are rarely the cause of your pain. More likely, the issue lies deeper and can be sourced somewhere in the spine – the pain is simply "referred" to the muscles. Use caution when following a muscle based therapy plan. Often prescribed solutions such as stretching will stimulate the stretch reflex and in doing so may feel good at the time but long term will create more damage to the spine underneath. Comprehensive testing is needed to determine your true source of pain. Only then can the issue be properly addressed.

Facet Joint Pathology: Facet joints guide movement and thus, when sensitized, cause pain with certain movements. The pain usually has a slower onset and can take several weeks to desensitize. This is assisted by identifying the painful spine movements and avoiding them – by moving about the hips instead.

Torn or Strained Ligaments: Ligaments can tear off the vertebral bones upon experiencing forced awkward joint postures such as those the body would be forced into in a martial arts submission hold. The ligaments themselves can also be torn in their midsection from impact loads such as those experienced in vehicle collisions. These damaged ligaments cause joint laxity and often result in long-term joint pain. By avoiding spine bending altogether through controlled movements and muscle stiffening, the joint can gristle and stabilize itself over time – we may be talking over a year!

Scoliosis: This condition involves an unnatural side-to-side "S" shape curvature in the spine. This abnormal shape of the spine can cause instability, disc bulges and pave the way for other injuries if not managed properly. Sometimes people develop these curves during their growth years. I have written more extensively about the assessment and treatment using Schroth exercises which have assisted many challenging patients.

Muscle Inhibition: This feeling of immobility is often a byproduct of hip and back pain. Certain muscle groups become inhibited, others become facilitated and feel tight. Generally back pained individuals develop inhibited gluteal muscles (the buttocks) and psoas tightness (the large muscle that connects the spine and thigh). The tightness is felt in the crease between the leg and torso. This muscular imbalance causes further changes in how load is experienced in the joints of the hip and spine. Patients who experience muscle inhibition face an additional challenge on their way to becoming pain free but, like everything it can be dealt with. We will address specific healing techniques later.

Traumatic damage: Fractures and other traumatic tissue damage should be diagnosed with initial treatment from trauma specialists. Sometimes the damage is much more extensive than that visible on medical images (X-Rays, CT and MRI images). For example, movement engrams are the coded movements that form habitual movement patterns. These are stored in the motor cortex of the brain but also in the spinal cord itself. Sometimes during trauma the cord is "shocked" causing disruption of the engrams. For example I had a patient that could no longer perform a simple task such as crossing her legs after she was in an auto accident. Other times the perception of movement is mixed with pain perception so that syndromes such as fibromyalgia develop. The key for clinical success here is to begin with simple pain-free movement and slowly build the pain-free repertoire by over-writing the perturbed engrams.

A Word About the Aging Back

The nature of back pain is very age-dependent. If you ask an older person about back pain, they will often relate to symptoms they experienced in their thirties, forties and fifties but will remark that they have none now. Discogenic pain, the pain that originates from a damaged vertebral disc, is rampant among the young, yet rare among more senior citizens. The difference is that seniors who do experience back pain are more likely dealing with spine arthritis and stenosis (a narrowing of the spinal canal that pinches nerves). The bottom line is that age should always be taken into consideration when matching a pain trigger to a therapeutic activity, as often times older patients are dealing with a different set of issues.

Understanding Pain: Why do we "pick the scab"?

Many back pain sufferers would experience a huge breakthrough in their recovery if they only realized that it was their flawed movement patterns that kept them pain-sensitive. Much like a scab forming on our skin, our backs our constantly trying to patch and heal themselves. We, however, by continuing to repeat harmful movement patterns in our daily lives cause re-injury. We are essentially "picking the scab." It is unreasonable to expect the body to heal if we continue to provoke it in the same way that led to the original injury. Continued provocation of pain sensitizes the nerves so that pain is triggered with even less stimulation. Remove the provocative motions and we can find the solution.

Here's how pain sensitivity works: people increase their sensitivity through repeated stressful and painful loading. The muscles and joints are loaded with sensors: pain sensors, pressure sensors, force sensors, chemical sensors. Some detect carbon dioxide, some detect pain, some sense histamine for inflammation. Human joints are packed with sensors that relay position and movement information to the brain. These signals travel along the sensory nerves. Along the highway of nerves there are checkpoints, or "gates", at junctions. According to the Gate Theory of Pain, the idea is, to flood the checkpoint with "good information", in other words signals associated with pain-free movement. In this way there is no more room for the pain signals as they are crowded out.

Try this: close your eyes and find the tip of your nose with your finger like in a roadside sobriety test. You are using kinesthetic sensory organs that run throughout your arm to navigate. These sensors alert the brain as to the position of your forefinger in relation to your nose. The sensation of this simple pain-free motion dominates the information traffic on your sensory nerves with feel-good kinesthetic sensory information that identifies position, length and force. ***Finding and repeating pain-free motions in your back will cause the remaining painful activities to hurt less. Read the previous sentence again – it really is that important.***

By discovering and engraining positive movements for your back, you will find that the pain often dissipates and then disappears entirely. This is because when we remove pain triggers and stop "picking the scab" we give our tissues a chance to rest, heal and regenerate. Simultaneously our sensors for pain are actually being desensitized. Master this, and you have mastered your back pain.

What is Psychosomatic Pain?

Although many patients are wrongly dismissed by their doctors for having psychosomatic pain (meaning it's all in their heads), it is true that certain individuals are prone to magnifying their pain. This is not because the patient is mentally unstable but it may be that they are a perfectionist. I find I am able to identify these types of patients very early into an initial interview. They get annoyed when their body is not functioning perfectly. They tend to be detail oriented and have more "driven" personalities. One of their major fears is that their back trouble will cause them to lose their hard-earned fitness. They want to know the exact date they can return to challenging training. Does this sound like you?

Or perhaps you fit into another category of patient who tends to be more focused specifically on the ache – they obsess over their pain. For these individuals, finding something else to focus on can be a helpful tool. Many of them have been told by a pain clinic to record their pain levels on a scale every day, which forces them to dwell on the pain!

If you fall into either of the above categories you need to find a tool to mentally deal with your pain as you follow the steps to recovering physically. ***When you experience pain throughout the day, instead of obsessing over it, acknowledge that you***

feel it and use this as a reminder to adjust your postures and movement patterns. By focusing on the solution, rather than the problem, your recovery will be much more productive.

The Degenerative Cascade

Let's contrast a back injury with the principles of healing a broken leg. In the case of the leg, let's say a broken fibula, the bone will eventually form a callous and heal stronger than the original bone. The joints remain healthy and no residual consequences remain. A back injury is different in the sense that spine tissues do not heal in a matter of weeks. Instead, the damage and altered spine joint mechanics cause a chain reaction or "cascade" of issues that may last years. For example, an original injury in the spine endplate, may lead to a disc bulge, which will result in a flatter disc and narrowed joint space, which in turn may trap a nerve root. The flattened space then places more load on the posterior facet joints that then respond by developing arthritis over the following two years. Thus, motion becomes more painful as the new arthritic bone growth gnaws away at the nerve roots. Micro-movements of the spine only continue to cause more irritation. Confused yet?

The essence of this information is that the natural degenerative cascade that can occur after a single back injury or condition is common but can be managed. The cascade may continue for a time internally, but the pain can be lessened and even eliminated with posture change and movement control. Successful patients will be able to "manage" their back pain over a period of time to ensure it doesn't worsen. If a joint injury is properly managed over approximately ten years, the unavoidable cascade will continue, but the pain is successfully managed. Then the joint will stiffen on its own and the pain will eventually subside and disappear.

Chapter Summary

A great deal of very technical information has been presented in this chapter and I hope I haven't overwhelmed you. By establishing many of these basic principles now, you will be able to better understand the concepts in the chapters that follow. Let's do a quick review.

It is important to remember that in order to heal your back you need to be able to recognize what is triggering your pain. Understanding the basics of back anatomy, posture and movement, as well as specific types of injuries will all help you identify ways to avoid your pain. You can then discern between the helpful and the damaging courses of action. We will devise specific action plans for you later in the book.

For those of you that have a known type of injury, a name to attach to your condition, your personal recovery strategy should always begin with avoiding the original pain-inducing mechanism. Focusing on avoiding the aggravating posture for your unique spine is key to getting yourself back on track.

Various symptoms of back pain have a distinct and known cause (although this information is not widely known making this book uniquely valuable). Injuries can be avoided if we avoid the injury mechanism itself. Here's a recap of some pain avoidance strategies, as well as an introduction of some that will be discussed later. The knowledge in this chapter will provide the foundation that will help you:

1. Locate and eliminate the cause of your pain – get an appropriate assessment that provides a specific diagnosis (you will be able to obtain your own by reading chapter 6).
2. Increase your consciousness around what movements and postures cause you pain.
3. Develop replacement postures and movement patterns that enable you to function pain-free.
4. Stabilize your torso, core and spine to remove painful spine joint micro-movements.
5. Develop a daily exercise plan that includes walking.
6. Mobilize your hips.
7. Learn to create power at the ball and socket joints (hips and shoulders).

8. Learn exercises that are based on patterns of movement: push, pull, lift, carry, lunge, squat etc.
9. Make healthy spine choices when sleeping, sitting, or engaging in more demanding activities.

You're on your way to learning the secrets of a pain-free lifestyle! Let's make it happen!

Chapter 3

Is Surgery for You? – the Essential List

Is Surgery for You? – the Essential List

Ninety-five percent of the challenging patients I see do NOT need surgery, even though many were told that was their only cure. My opinion is based on my three decades of experience, working with patients who have been successful with surgical avoidance and in dealing with the "failed backs" caused by "unsuccessful" surgery. At my clinic, we follow-up with every patient to keep "score", so, we know who got better.

After having surgery, the patient is forced to rest. Ironically, this post-surgery recuperation is often as effective in pain reduction as the actual surgery itself. Let the following statement really sink in: *In many cases, had the patient subjected themselves to the rest associated with the surgery – and skipped the surgery – the results would have been just as good.*

Surgery constitutes "rolling the dice". There is no "undo" button. Essential nerve and muscle tissue is cut. The scarring process that ensues sometimes grabs onto nerves, resulting in potentially chronic back pain. Essential bone is removed creating a permanent loss: in these areas of the body bone does *not* grow back.

Surgery does work for some people. But beware. It may work for only a period of time. Studies show that initial progress may be made but that after a few years, the surgical patient's status is comparable to those who chose the non-surgical option. The major reason for this is that the original flawed mechanics that lead to the tissue breakdown and resulting pain were never addressed. The operated site stabilized but now the level above or below has experienced the same damage. Essentially, if a symptom is surgically "cured" but the cause is never addressed, the symptom will reappear in another area. Surgery, without rehabilitation to change the flawed movement patterns rarely creates a permanent solution. My advice to you is this: if you are considering surgery don't rush. Follow the steps in this chapter and you will achieve the most informed, low risk and successful approach over the longer term.

Try "Virtual Surgery"

Patients who have tried physical therapy, Pilates, chiropractic and traction therapy, among countless other techniques, are frequently told that surgery is their only remaining option. Here is an approach I recommend to them. First, I doubt that any of these therapies addressed the real cause of their pain. I ask them if they have been thoroughly assessed and whether the pain causing movements, postures and loads have been identified. The majority of them share the same answer – "No".

I respond by saying, "Before we do any rehabilitation we are going to play the 'virtual surgery game'. This means I will lead you through the recovery program of a surgery patient without actually going under the knife. Today, let's pretend I gave you surgery. This means that you will not go to the gym or stretch tomorrow. You will rest. We will, very slowly and methodically, build a progressive rehabilitation program for you." The recovery program would follow the principles outlined in this book. They include:

- Erasing the cause of pain
- Establishing pain-free movement patterns
- Walking
- Some specific exercises.

I am convinced that some surgeries work for no other reason than they have forced the patient to take the time to rest. Always try this approach before going ahead with an actual surgical procedure. Many of my patients have done better than the statistical outcome for surgery, by employing these techniques alone.

When looking at surgery, consider the following:

- First, always try the "virtual surgery" approach and consider surgery only when it fails.

- Surgery should be considered when neurological issues are substantial such as loss of bowel or bladder control.

- Radiating pain symptoms, numbness, muscle atrophy, etc. are all signs of trapped or compromised spine nerve roots. We have been successful in each of these conditions using nerve mobilization approaches together with mechanically based movement therapy. Always try these first. Caution: These are special techniques that require expertise. Performed improperly or too aggressively they will increase symptoms. Approaches to reduce the cause of the nerve compression or irritation are also required in the more stubborn cases (see the chapter on nerve flossing).

- Surgery may be considered in cases of trauma. Broken bone and torn tissues often need stabilizing.

- Pain must be unrelenting and severe for a substantial period of time before surgery is to be considered. Patients who have severe pain for as little as three weeks and then have surgery have been some of the most disabled post-surgical cases I have seen.

- If you have good and bad days in terms of pain, you are not a surgery candidate. You do need to identify the cause of the changing pain.

- Beware of "new" treatments. Over three decades I have observed many "new devices" that have been surgically put into people that do not meet expectations over the long term. Discs have been stiffened with papain injections, heated with a catheter to stiffen them, cored and screwed with various implants, to name a few. None of these lived up to initial claims and expectations.

- Disc replacement is another approach that I am very sceptical of. I have not seen a long term "successful" case yet – success being defined as the full resumption of former activities without pain. Most spine joint pain results from motion and loading. Traditionally the surgeons "fuse" the joint in a variety of ways. But an artificial disc does the opposite. Its goal is to restore motion to the joint. But herein lies the flaw. The disc is just one of three joints at each spine level. The artificial disc creates an axis of rotation that rarely mimics the natural axes of the natural disc. This places more stress on the other two facet joints. Over time, they become arthritic and intolerant to motion. Long-term spine health is very difficult to achieve using this approach.

- Always exhaust the conservative options. You may think that because you tried "physical therapy" or some other approach once and it failed, that surgery is your only option. There may be other therapies that are more appropriate for you.

- Beware of the "institutes" that offer to view your scans (CT, MRI) and advise you on their surgery options, without assessing YOU. They are assuming that the picture shows the pain and that they can cut the pain out. My science and experience suggests that in many cases, the pain is actually coming from a structure that looks fine on the MRI image while the nasty looking disc is really pain-free. A surgeon must confirm that the pain is indeed coming from the structure identified in the MRI. Having stated this, an MRI can sometimes reveal injury mechanisms through linking distinct patterns of tissue damage. My advice is to avoid a medical service provider who does not conduct an extensive examination of the patient.

When selecting the surgeon:

- Take this matter into your own hands. Everyone likes to say that they had the best surgeon. I have seen some I would not let put a screw into my basement wall – they are that sloppy and uncaring. Just because a surgeon is the head of the department or they spoke at a medical conference, this does not directly translate to the skill in their hands. I have found that asking the nurses and physical therapists at the hospital which surgeon has the best results is a wise approach.

- Some surgeons state, "Everyone does well with this surgery." There is no surgery that is without risk nor is there one that always produces a good outcome. Clarify what the "success rate" of the operation is. The word "success" can be loaded. In some medical reports this means the patient did not die. In others, it means that the patient did well for a brief period of time following the operation. You are most interested in the longer term success rate compared to any other option, and with a balanced understanding of both the risks and benefits. Obtain the long term results.

- If hip surgery is their main focus and spine surgery comprises only a small part of their surgeries I suggest that you find another surgeon. It takes a lot of practice to become competent in operating on the spine. Find a surgeon who has performed the procedure many times, many hundreds of times is even better!

- There are some surgeons who state, "I always do the neck first and then do the back." This surgery "up-selling" sounds ridiculous but it happens. It is highly unlikely that a patient would have operable anatomic lesions in both the neck and back. If you hear this, I suggest you look for another surgeon.

- If a surgeon proposes doing a multilevel fusion in the lumbar spine for degenerative disc disease I strongly suggest you look elsewhere. The spine is meant to move. Although fusing one or possibly two levels for a badly degenerated disc is reasonable, fusing multiple levels rarely is necessary or advisable.

- A good surgeon always discusses options, alternatives and the risk/reward. If the surgeon does not offer you any non-surgical treatment options they may be operating under the old *"I have a hammer so I will treat everything as a nail"* adage.

- If the surgeon becomes perturbed by you asking questions, you must find another surgeon. A well-qualified and informed physician does not mind a patient asking questions, most encourage it. A marginal physician is more likely to be put out by an inquisitive patient.

- You must avoid the surgeon who claims that he has never done this particular type of surgery but would like to try it. Don't be a guinea pig.

- When the first surgery does not work you must be very skeptical when the surgeon proposes doing it all over again. The most common reason a surgery does not work is that the patient did not need the surgery in the first place. The chance of a second surgery working is much lower.

Essential points to discuss with the surgeon:

- Ask the surgeon to set up a conversation with a couple of his former patients so you can be assured of their satisfaction.

- Discuss the pain with the surgeon. Determine what is the pain generator and can he cut it out? If there are several tissues involved, the chances for success go down. If there is damage at several spine levels then the chance for success drops substantially. If your doctor cannot clearly articulate the anatomic problem and how they will correct it, I strongly suggest you find another surgeon.

A Typical Story: Make sure that it is not about you and failed surgery

Your strategy to obtain the best outcome is to follow the rules above. Considering surgery is serious business.

Here is an all-too-typical tale of back woe: a person goes to the family doctor with back pain. The family doctor not knowing how to address the cause writes a prescription, (the family doctor sees the patient is obviously pained so they prescribe pain medication). If the pain persists they might suggest a surgical consultation or refer the pained patient to a physical therapist.

The pained patient may be referred to a surgeon. The surgeon says, "Indeed, there is a problem and I can fix it with surgery." A surgical date is set and quite often during the waiting time the patient will get better. The back pain goes away on its own. The confused patient has no idea what they did to cure the pain and is equally perplexed as to how to prevent future back pain attacks. But the pain will reoccur.

The unknowing (and now confused) patient gets better but still questions, "Should I go through with the surgery? Do I not have the surgery? What to do?"

One likely diagnosis a good back professional might make is that the discogenic back pain (disc pain) is episodic. By episodic we mean, a really nasty attack occurs and then goes away, repeating the cycle again and again.

Our ill-informed patient again sees the surgeon. "Doc, I felt better after I last saw you and I was pain-free for three months. But, then I picked up a bag of groceries the wrong way and had a relapse. That was two weeks ago, but I feel good now. What do you think?"

The patient gets a whole five minutes of the surgeon's precious time. Some surgeons may say, "Since it is reoccurring, why don't we go through with the surgery and be done with all this episodic stuff." On the other hand the surgeon seeing that this patient is not an absolute emergency case they might suggest something very inappropriate, "Why don't we put off the surgery and why don't you try Yoga or Pilates?"

What goes wrong

The flaw in logic and process here is that the surgeon failed to proceed to an assessment of the pain triggers. Frankly the majority of them are not trained in these skills. Most likely, the triggers will also be present in Yoga or Pilates exercises. The fundamental flaw is this: an episodically pained patient is not a surgical case. The fact that they have pain-free days shows they simply need to identify the triggers that cause a painful day and eliminate them.

Every back-pained patient should ask the questions outlined above. Most don't. Doing your own sleuth work beforehand may help you to avoid becoming another case in the long list of unfortunate people who have undergone surgery only to experience partial healing, or worse, "the failed and desperate back." These patients opted to go the surgery route only to experience disappointing results. Many are worse now than they were before the procedure.

Final Thoughts

In a perfect world, the back-pained patient commits to a justifiable and progressive remedial journey that is active in the best sense of the word. The patient becomes an educated active participant in his or her own therapy. Patients are guided by competent clinicians who do not provide the same therapy to every patient. Instead, health practitioners work to understand and assess the individual and directly address the cause of that individual's pain. Anything less provides opportunity for poor practice to continue.

The best chance you have of challenging status quo is to: arm yourself with information; ask the tough questions; hold your health practitioners to a higher standard; focus on assessment and proper identification of your unique back issues; and then take an active role on the path to achieving back health. In other words, you need to take the steps required to become your own back mechanic.

Chapter 4

The Code: Rules and Guidelines for Back Health

The Code
Rules and Guidelines for Back Health

Successfully avoiding future back pain, managing current pain and achieving full potential from your back requires that you adhere to the "code," that is, the "code" required for a resilient back and a pain-free lifestyle.

As Captain Barbosa stated in that famous line in the film "Pirates of the Caribbean" upon reneging his deal with Elizabeth, "Ah, the Pirate's code – they're more like guidelines!" The following principles aren't the absolute rules for recovery but rather a set of wise guidelines intended to be adaptable to you.

Here are some guidelines that form the code for achieving better back health.

Guideline # 1: Dedicate yourself to practicing healthful back activity everyday.

Appropriate movement positively influences the health of every body system. Make a conscious effort to engage in healthy movement every day, and soon enough this will become habit.

Guideline # 2: Get the big picture right - maintain balance.

You will achieve optimal health and healing by creating a balance of appropriate sleep, good diet, and a matched activity/training program. Those who fail to recognize the importance of this balance will continue to rob Peter to pay Paul. Peter is opportunity and Paul is a lead weight dragging you down and thwarting your progress.

Guideline # 3: Remove the cause. Avoid painful and weakened postures.

There is a direct correlation between posture, position and pain. Avoiding painful and weakened postures is one of my paramount principles. Prepare the spine to bear load successfully by seeking and maintaining neutral spine posture.

Common sense corollary guideline # 3: if certain postures and movements induce pain, identify these painful and weakened postures and avoid them!

The trick is in performing "spine hygiene". This means moving well throughout the day, avoiding painful movements, expanding your pain-free repertoire of activity capacity, and building some capacity for corrective exercise. In other words, what you don't do is just as important, if not more, as what you *do* do.

Guideline # 4: Beware of clinicians whose "treatments" require numerous return visits.

If you are injured and in pain and seek professional help, expect the competent expert to address and heal the problem within a reasonable amount of time. If a clinician's expertise lies in relieving pain without curing the cause of the pain, the patient ends up seeing the clinician repeatedly. While repeat visits are good for the clinicians business, they do nothing (other than possibly offering temporary relief) to address the overriding issue. The best clinicians see you fewer times, as they teach you how to take responsibility for your healing, and give you the tools to do so.

Guideline # 5: Be aware of "passive treatments".

Treatment falls into two broad categories:

- Passive treatment: designed to cure the pain (the symptom)
- Active treatment: designed to address and cure the cause

Passive treatment is having somebody do something to you. For example having an ultrasound machine rubbed over your back is passive treatment: the patient simply sits; stands or lies down while someone does something to the patient. Passive therapies administered from devices do not address or correct the cause of the pain. Passive treatment rarely increases the likelihood of a long-term back pain cure. In contrast, there is occasion where passive approaches such as certain chiropractic manipulations, or muscle based treatments address part of the cause. They can enable a window of opportunity to enjoy a period of pain-free movement. But they must be combined with active patient engagement in enhancing movement quality to cure a patient.

Active treatment requires the patient to participate in some manner or fashion that works toward a cure. For example, learning to move in a way that avoids the pain triggers is an active treatment. Avoid becoming an ATM machine for ineffectual or incompetent clinicians: reserve your right to walk away if the clinician focuses all their efforts on relief and none on cure.

Guideline # 6: Buyer beware – not all clinicians are competent.

Many back pain sufferers presume all clinicians are competent. Just as there are good auto mechanics and bad auto mechanics, good professors and terrible ones, there are good clinicians and poor ones. Patients tend to place medical professionals on a pedestal and a few will use this to their advantage. They adopt authoritarian attitudes that subtly or overtly imply, "How dare you ask questions about my professional methods!" But the patient is the consumer, you have full right to question why, and how a particular treatment plan is best for you.

Ultrasound, for example, a very popular passive technique, has never been shown to cure back disorders better than placebo. Surgery rarely cures the individual if after the surgery the patient continues to repeat the faulty movement patterns that caused the original disorder. I believe it should be legislated that no surgery can proceed until the mechanical cause of the pain has been shown to the patient – I will coach you to find the cause in the next chapter. There is no question that some soft tissue treatments such as trigger-point therapy, Active Release Technique and topflight chiropractic treatment *can* assist in a fully successful program – assuming the treatments are few in number and they are combined with active treatments.

Guideline # 7: If you've left the Doctor's office with only pain pills and no plan for active treatment, you did not see a back expert.

Truth be known, many family doctors admit they don't know what to do with back pain patients. They mean well, however, prescribing pain medications is what they know. Unfortunately, patients who have pharmaceutically numbed their pain often make matters worse in that they are able to continue using flawed and perturbed movement patterns. This makes a bad situation worse.

You need to know what a good movement pattern is before you can start prescribing it. There is nothing in the training of family doctors that provides insight into the world of cutting-edge back health.

Guideline # 8: Establish the subtle balance between strength, power and endurance, mobility and stiffness.

If you add too much strength, you can "overpower" your back. The counterbalance for too much back strength and power is *endurance and control*. Endurance enables you to maintain perfect movement patterns as you get fatigued, repetition after repetition. Injury occurs when the perfect movement form is lost, causing stress and pain. Spine conserving movement requires spine stiffness (or firmness), coordinated with the centered motion of the hips and shoulders.

Guideline # 9: One therapeutic size does NOT fit all!

We all are unique creatures; we all have different backs and different hips that influence the back. The idea that a single magical exercise program exists that can be used in every instance is a ridiculous myth. Too often medical professionals and physical therapists use a single mode or method for every single patient regardless of individualized circumstance. While that is easy and convenient for the doctor or therapist, it is disastrous for the patient.

It is critical that the healthcare provider delve deeply into the patient's injury history and create a customized remedial strategy:

- The first order of business is to make the right functional diagnosis – determine the motions, postures and loads that cause the pain.
- The second is to remove the cause.
- The third step is to choose the appropriate rehabilitative strategy that includes movements that avoid pain and heal damaged tissue.
- The fourth order of business is to enhance and broaden pain-free activities.

Be aware that there are fundamental patterns of movement. This book is loaded with guidelines for pain-free ways to sit, walk, lift, drive, sleep and live life. If you seek professional guidance to help execute this plan, demand determination, care, great attention to finding the cause, the corrective starting points, create logical progressions of exercises and select an appropriate dosage. Upon completion of this book, however, most will be able to successfully direct their own plan.

Guideline # 10: Success is achieved through continued personal re-assessment.

As recovery progresses, the program must evolve. Pain-free movement patterns will expand, as will the "dose" of the training. Your pain-free tolerance will increase. The objective is to create training regimens that operate below the threshold that causes pain. If your training session leads to pain, you've done too much, too soon. Thus, the first stage of a program should be directed towards reducing pain. Subsequent stages are designed following re-assessment to increase pain-free activity.

Consider the case: The patient can find very few pain-free activities. Getting up out of a chair and walking five steps might be painless however six steps causes pain. Hence, their current pain capacity is five steps.

In this particular instance, the individual's five-step pain capacity is so low that it is not feasible for them to work with a rehabilitative specialist. The patient does not have sufficient pain tolerance. One method for increasing this particular individual's pain tolerance capacity is a commonsense approach: every hour get up and walk five pain-free steps. Slowly, over time, the patient will build capacity and be able to walk six steps, then seven, then eight and so on. Once the patient is able to walk say twenty steps, we might begin walks up and down the patient's driveway every hour. When the driveway is no longer challenging, walk around the block three times per day. The work/rest ratio changes to fewer, but more demanding sessions. The progression is guided by taking stock and reviewing progress through each stage.

We have now reviewed the guidelines that form the code! Simply put, as you take your own journey away from back pain and toward back health, the more of these guidelines you can follow, the more successful you will be.

Part Two:
Self-Assessment: Finding the cause of your pain

Why do people move in ways that are hurtful? Why do people sit, stand and move using postures and motions that cause or amplify the pain? I have wondered about the irony of this phenomenon. I suspect they move using painful movement patterns out of pure ingrained habit. In fact, this is why they remain pained.

What situations, movements and actions stress the spine? To know them (flawed movement patterns) is to know how to avoid them.

Here is a generalized approach to find the cause of pain. Only then can we devise an effective approach to eliminate it.

Chapter 5

Using the McGill Approach to Find Your Pain Trigger

Using the McGill Approach to Find Your Pain Trigger

Why do people sit, stand and engage in postures and motions that cause or amplify their pain? I have wondered about the irony of this phenomenon: injured and pained people seem drawn towards moving in ways that increase the level of pain. I suspect they continue to use these movement patters out of pure ingrained habit.

A big part of our clinical success can be attributed to identifying the cause of pain followed by creating customized, alternative pain-free movement patterns. To know these flawed movements is to know how to avoid them.

What I do and How the Approach Works

Here is the process I follow with each back-pained individual who visits my clinic/laboratory at the University. A typical appointment begins with using logical observation to make an initial visual assessment. How does the patient enter the room? Specifically, is there any telltale distortion in their walking pattern? How do they sway as they walk? Does one foot fall harder than the other? How does the back-pained patient sit down and rise out of their chair? Like a forensic detective looking for clues at a crime scene, I am keenly observing and searching for any and all visual tips and clues.

Early on in my career, I realized that I saw things that traditionally trained doctors were not seeing. This was because of my scientific training and I suppose, mechanical aptitude. I have had the opportunity to work alongside the great clinicians such as Drs Dick Erhard, Vladamir Janda, Shirley Sahrmann, and Clayton Skaggs. Each one had a keen eye and tremendous skill in recognizing patterns. I worked to hone a similar skill.

Here's an example. A couple of decades ago, a patient walked into an exam room where a surgeon and I were to examine him. From simple observation, I said to the surgeon, *"This man has nerve pressure on the 4th lumbar root on the right hand side. He has a posterior lateral disc bulge at that level. But it will be relieved by posture change and will not need surgery. Please have a look."*

The surgeon actually laughed and said, ***"That's a bold snap judgment."*** His dismissive disdain turned into wonderment when he examined the patient and found there to be a bulging disk precisely where I had indicated. ***"How could you have possibly known that?"*** He looked at me like I had just performed some baffling sleight-of-hand magic card trick. In actuality, I had used a process of pattern recognition, scientific logic, and deductive reasoning to determine the patient's maladies.

I could "hear" and "see" the patient's afflictions. I could hear the asymmetry when he walked; in this case, his right foot fell harder giving a subtle foot slap. I concluded that the muscle responsible for holding the foot up was not working due to a trapped nerve associated with the 4th lumbar root. As he strode into the room and took a seat, I noted he activated his hamstring muscles as a substitute for his inhibited gluteal muscles. Not overly, but subtly, barely noticeable – but it was there for the trained eye to see. I was able to make this observation based on our investigations, which have documented common patterns of how pain inhibits these muscles. These clues were there all along, as were a few more. Naturally the surgeon was astounded.

In my opinion, many medical doctors have become numb to their patients' displays of their pain. They develop a reserve and distance and purposefully will not engage in lengthy conversations with pain-afflicted individuals for a variety of reasons. One huge rationale is lack of time. There are substantial time pressures resulting from having patients lined up in a crowded waiting room. Another characteristic develops from the process of medical specialization which dulls the ability to process clues emitted from the entire body. For all these reasons they simply cannot "study" the patient.

These observations have two quite astounding implications: in most situations, you can become better at addressing your back pain than your doctor, and, you can be guided in the interpretation of your signs. I will show you how to study yourself, and devise a solution.

After I have noted these initial observations from the patient, I conduct an in-depth interview. A great deal of information can be learned by asking well-chosen questions and really listening to the answers as the back-pained patient describes how they got to this point. By the end of the interview I will have identified the activities that make the pain worse, the activities that are well tolerated, the patterns of pain progression throughout the day, and the nature of the pain, its locations, sensations, and radiating patterns.

With this information I create a hypothesis as to what should be avoided and what is tolerable. I then have the patient go through some physical tests. I am looking to find those movement patterns that cause pain and those movement patterns that bypass the pain. My goal is to identify, then share with the patient, pain-free alternative movement patterns. The movement patterns I recommend will cause the back less stress and in turn allow traumatized tissue the break needed to rest, heal and grow. Nature, in its infinite wisdom, is designed to heal the body given the right conditions.

By the time the back-pained patient leaves the consult I will have provided them with a two-stage plan: first they will get a series of pain-free alternative movements; and second a plan to add some therapeutic exercises as the pain sensitivity winds down. Too many clinicians simply provide resistance-building exercises for the patient. In bypassing the more delicate recovery phase that removes the cause of pain, they often cause further damage to the patient's fragile tissues and actually worsen their condition.

Now that we've covered a typical evaluation you would experience if you were to come see me in person, it's time we examine the at-home assessment you can perform on yourself!

Chapter 6

Your Self-Assessment

Your Self-Assessment

So far we have established that there is no such thing as "non-specific" back pain. Something is causing the pain, and once identified, we refer to the pain as specific. We have also established that repeated irritation of painful tissues only makes them more sensitive. The irritation comes from poor movement and postures coupled with unnecessary stresses. These are the pain triggers. Your task is to detect and identify your personal triggers and eliminate them.

A detailed spine pain assessment requires the skills of an expert diagnostician. That being said, only a few back pain sufferers will need this level of expertise and assessment. This chapter will guide you through the process of diagnosing the cause of your pain. Remember there is no doctor who can understand or measure your pain better than you can yourself. In many cases you will be the best diagnostician for your own back pain!

Let's get started. I suggest you read this chapter in its entirety, then get a notebook, set aside some time, get comfortable and read through it once again. This second time through, physically proceed through these diagnostic exercises one by one, and record your findings. You may require some assistance with a few of them, so you might consider having someone on standby that can help when required.

We begin by ensuring that there are no "sinister" reasons (such as a tumor) for your pain. Then we will follow a process to identify your pain triggers. The goal, of course, is that you will be able to reach a precise diagnosis in terms of the triggers of your pain. I will then guide you through the process of addressing your triggers in the final chapters. For the few of you who are unable to find the triggers, I have provided a set of guidelines to find the best medical people who will conduct an assessment to guide your recovery.

The Essential Precaution

First, you must eliminate the possibility that there is a sinister cause of your back pain. This is rare. The process begins with a visit to your primary care physician who is trained to interpret various signs and results. Your physician should include in the review: blood test results, recent unintentional changes in weight, any history of trauma, bowel or bladder incontinence, cancer, intravenous drug use, systemic illness, back pain with fever, progressive and constant night pain, abdominal pain (particularly between the navel and pubis), and saddle anesthesia which is numbness around your inner thighs and pelvic floor. In addition, your doctor will be able to eliminate the possibility of restricting vascular and cardiac conditions so that you are clear to partake in a physical rehabilitation program.

Very rarely, I found sinister causes that were not detected in the physicians screening process. Generally these people's back pains were unresponsive to changes in spine motions, postures, and loads. Their pain was unrelenting as they were not able to reduce their pain with posture and movement change during the assessment. They were directed back to the physician who delved deeper to find the cause.

Some Context for the Assessment

The typical orthopedic exam would begin with determining the patient's range of spine motion, or perhaps commence with neurological measures of strength or reflexes, or even tests of maximum muscle strength. This does little to identify the cause of pain.

Other doctors walk into the exam room and their first move is to put the MRI or CT images on the viewing screen. They declare what the "problem" is, or isn't. The physical exam lasts all of five minutes. No patient deserves this treatment, but it is all too common. Our goal is to custom design a prevention and rehabilitation program for every patient regardless of his or her situation.

A few years back we tracked the progress of back pain patients who were going to a particular pain clinic. We recorded their initial patient scores for range of motion and back strength and then followed up over the next few months to see how they progressed. The scores obtained from the initial assessment were not predictive of who got better. There appears to be a disconnect between what is traditionally assessed and what is helpful for predicting future pain, or reducing current pain. This is what we do know:

- Movement that begins from the spine predicts a poor future for back pain. For example, the person who moves with their spine first (as apposed to their hips or shoulders), when reaching to open a door needs movement training.
- Certain asymmetries of strength and movement have been shown to be predictive of current or future back troubles.
- Stiff hips, particularly on one side is a good predictor of future back disorders.
- Tight hamstring muscles are not very predictive of future disorders. However, asymmetry between right and left sides is a bit more predictive power for future pain.
- Imbalance in torso muscle endurance is highly problematic, particularly when the back muscle endurance scores are poorer than the scores for the abdominal muscles.
- Pain induced with prolonged sitting and standing usually predicts more intense pain in the future.

Our approach in identifying the cause of pain during an assessment is to intentionally provoke it. Provocative pain testing is essential and irreplaceable when it comes to determining which postures, motions, and loads trigger and amplify pain and which ones offer pain-free movement alternatives. These alternate movements and motions allow the individual to enjoy a pain-free life and wind down the pain sensitivity so that what may have hurt last month is found to be tolerable next month.

Let's guide you through finding and removing your personal pain triggers.

Administer Your Own Self-examination

Step 1 - Questions to help you hone in on the cause: Make your lists

First, get a piece of paper and write down all the activities that you have found to increase your back pain throughout the day. Then on a second list, write down a list of activities that do not increase your back pain and those that you can perform pain-free. Now examine and compare the two lists. Is there a common motion, posture, or load among the activities that cause pain? If so, you are beginning to zero in on your personal problem area. For example, if sitting for more than 15 minutes, tying your shoes in the morning and driving a car are activities that increase pain, yet walking does not cause pain, the pain mechanism is posture, specifically a flexed spine posture. In this specific case, we refer to the pain mechanism as "flexion intolerance" (recall figure in chapter 2 showing spine flexion).

Another example obtained from your lists would be that pain starts after five minutes of walking and increases with duration. However, you find that sitting, lying down, or having traction forces applied to your legs relieves the pain. If you are older, say more than 55, chances are your spine is arthritic. You will find relief with certain approaches that will restore walking ability in short intervals, slowly increasing the duration over time.

Next, continue the self-examination process with a few fundamental questions that will provide the clues we need to help in selecting a healing approach.

The Essential Questions

1. ***Does the pain change in intensity?*** Do you ever have a pain-free morning or at least a few hours? If your pain changes, there is a reason. Understanding the reason guarantees success. We will teach you how to identify the causes of your pain.
2. ***When you roll over in bed do you encounter painful "catches?"*** If you answered yes then you may have spinal instability. You may also experience painful stabs or shots when moving, such as reaching into the car trunk, or even when sneezing. These are further signs of instability. You can eliminate these stabs by stiffening your back with stabilization exercises shown later. They prevent the painful micro-motions of the spinal joints

that trigger pain sensors. Other activities to avoid include spine manipulation (such as a chiropractic treatment), spine stretching exercises and many of the commonly prescribed back exercises that involve bending and twisting, such as the scorpion exercise (lying on your back with the knees bent, then dropping the knees side to side twisting the spine – never do this when you have pain).

3. ***What makes your pain worse?*** If you are able to state any specific activity, then the pain has a specific trigger. The solution is found in avoiding the specific trigger. If managed carefully and properly, you won't have to cut a pleasurable activity such as golf or biking out of your life entirely, you will merely have to make adjustments to your movement patterns while partaking, in order to eliminate the specific trigger. As an example, does the pain only occur when engaged in a specific activity such as pickup basketball? Or, squatting with a barbell on your shoulders? If so, you have a resilient back for daily living. However, you are replicating the injury mechanism in the more demanding pain-causing activity. These can be identified and eliminated through technique modification or avoidance. For example, beware of spine flexion at the bottom of a squat – even the slightest amount will trigger disc pain in those sensitized with a disc bulge. Heavy breathing during basketball allows the spine to lose protective joint stiffness. This may be addressed with corrective breathing exercises – all shown later.

4. ***Was the initial cause of pain traumatic?*** A car accident or a fall perhaps? Or was the pain onset slow and undefinable – does the pain continue to worsen? Pain from a traumatic incident will likely be "mechanical" in nature meaning that pain reducing postures and movements should still be available.

5. ***Do you have any history of conditions such as osteoporosis?*** If so, there will be general fragility concerns with activity – choose exercise that spares the spine of compressive load. For example, when walking, try to maintain an upright posture, as bending forward will stress the spine with compression forces. These patients should avoid golf, which is an activity that stresses the spine but does not train muscle. Along with walking, swimming may be an exercise of choice for these individuals if the spine posture is not bent into deviated postures.

6. ***Is the pain at its worst, first thing in the morning?*** If so, bed choice may play a substantial role. Fine-tuning the stiffness of the mattress is likely part of the ultimate solution. For example, those with a large natural hollow in their low back, or who have more meat in the buttock area will not do well sleeping on a futon or hard, very firm mattress. This will cause their lumbar area to be unsupported when sleeping on the back resulting in morning pain and stiffness. A robust "pillow top" on top of the mattress often helps. Others adopt inappropriate sleeping postures such as the "fetal position" on the advice of others. This stresses the spinal discs keeping them sensitive. The solution is to find postures where the natural curves are maintained in the spine.

7. ***Does the pain increase throughout the day?*** If so, this pain pattern indicates that through the cumulative loading of your back, a point is reached where pain begins to present itself. From here, as loading continues, the pain worsens. All of us have a limit for pain-free loading. Pain that increases as your day continues, suggests that you are not practicing appropriate spine hygiene. The solution is to create a strategy that involves more spine conserving movement patterns together with "rest breaks" to restore some of the pain-free capacity. Just as an athlete "interval trains" to increase the tolerable volume of training, the back-pained individual needs "intervals" between loading of their body and rest. Several suggestions are provided later to accomplish this.

8. ***Is the pain more concentrated in your middle back?*** If so, begin by examining your default movement strategy if someone were to tell you to "sit up straight" from a slouched posture. This simple test will reveal if you are "hinging" at the thoracolumbar junction (rib cage and top of the lumbar spine) and focusing movement stress at the site of pain (this diagnostic test will be further explained later). Specific exercises can address this.

9. ***Does your back pain also radiate into your buttocks, legs and feet?*** This pain is almost always due to a trapped nerve root in the lumbar spine that is made worse with specific activity. The activity usually involves a deviated posture such as spine flexion that causes the disc bulge to grow and place pressure on the nerve. Other potential causes include arthritis in which the bone growth irritates the nerve root with direct compression or with movement. Again, more pristine movement usually reduces/eliminates the pain.

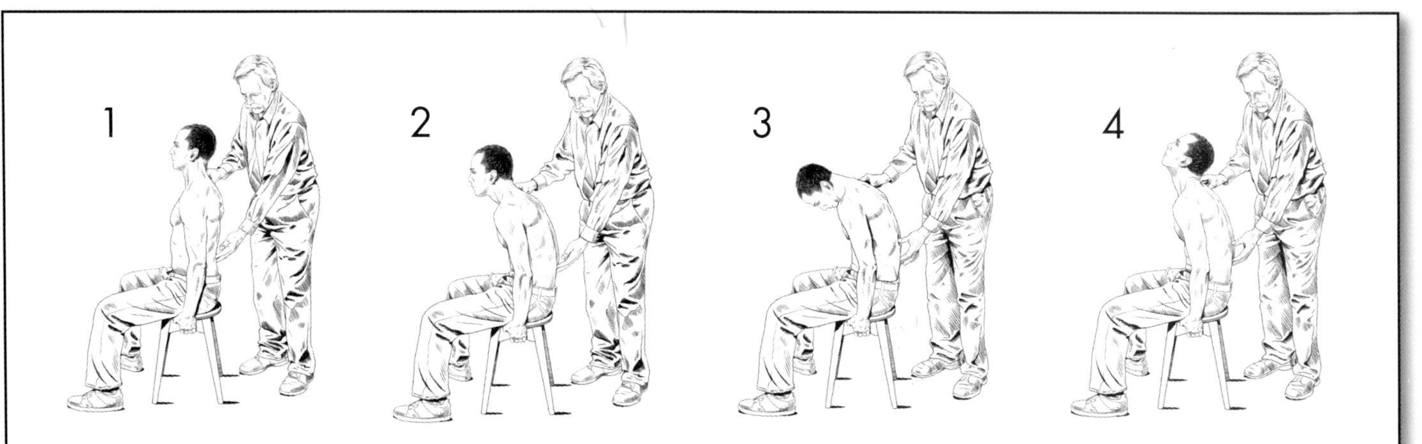

Test 1. (1) Pull up gently on the chair seat to add compressive load to your back. (2) Then flex the spine and repeat the pullup force to see if the pain sensitivity changes. (3) Maintain the slouched posture and flex the neck tightening the spinal nerves and repeat the pullup force. (4) Then extend the neck to relax the nerve tension and repeat. Then repeat the entire sequence with the spine in an extended posture noting what makes the pain better or worse.

10. ***Does the pain increase with fast walking or does it decrease?*** For those with pain from a disc bulge, slow walking, or "mall strolling", will increase low back pain. Yet fast walking (or "powerwalking") with your arms swinging about the shoulders will reduce pain, turning the original pain mechanism into a therapy. Those with stenosis, however, will find that walking simply adds to the cumulative load on their back, resulting in a slow windup of pain as the walking continues. In this case, a program of "corrected walking" to create a more spine-sparing style will help when combined with rest breaks – shown in the "walking" chapter.

Step 2 - Evaluate your lists

Let's compare again the two lists with the answers to the "essential questions". Let's see if we can narrow down some common features. Are the painful behaviors noted in the first list consistent with the answers? Do all the pain-causing activities have a common feature such as a specific spine posture, a particular movement, or a particular type of load or stress? Similarly, do the pain-free activities share a common activity such as walking?

The next step will help you hone in on specific pain triggers.

Step 3 - Evaluate your pain triggers with pain provocation and relieving tests

Here are some tests to reveal your pain triggers and help you find alternate pain-free strategies to sidestep these triggers. To be very clear, in the following tests, we are now purposefully trying to make the pain, or discomfort, worse. We do this to precisely identify the pain triggers. The three specific areas of potential triggers we will be examining are postures, loads and movements. Then, we will find ways to avoid the triggers and desensitize the pain-causing tissues.

Postures that make compression painful:

The following tests produce a minimal compressive load through the spine in order to help you identify your problem postures.

1. Sit on a stool and, with your arms at your side, grab the underside of the seat pan (Test 1). Sit-up tall so that your spine is in its neutral position. Pull up with your hands to compress the spine. Is this painful? Record your findings. Now repeat the pulling motion with the same intensity, but this time instead of sitting with a tall posture, allow yourself to slouch. Record your results in regards to pain. Finally, repeat the test one

more time with the spine in an extended (or "arched back") position. Document your results. If the tall posture test was painful, you have determined that spinal *compression* is a pain trigger for you. If the slouched sitting posture generated pain, spinal *flexion* is your pain trigger. If you found the spine extension painful, spinal *extension* is your primary trigger. If you have no pain in the tall posture but pain in slouched sitting, you have flexion based pain. Clearly your pain is a function of posture.

What is the most painful spine posture?____________________

What is the least painful spine posture?____________________

Now add neck, or cervical spine flexion (position 3) and extension (position 4) to each of the postures.

Is there more back pain in position 3?____________________

Is there more back pain in position 4?____________________

If you have more pain in position 3 than 4 then there is nerve tension pain, likely caused by a bulging disc or less likely some arthritic change. If position 4 is more painful you have a rare form of neural pain likely caused by a disc bulge "underhooking" a nerve (find a clinician familiar with my *Low Back Disorders* textbook). Now return to position 1 and repeat the sequence with the spine extended. If more pain is experienced then we have more follow-up tests to perform.

What do these results mean in terms of a solution? Simply put, if you remove the offending action from your repertoire of daily motions, you will effectively remove the cause of the pain. Because these four tests involve putting the spine under load, be extra conscious to avoid placing additional forces on your back when you find yourself using your pain-triggering posture. Certain back-pained patients will find that pain is caused in flexion *and* extension – for these there is just one position that is pain-free: neutral. These patients must try and avoid deviating from a neutral position whenever possible during their recovery. One movement tool particularly helpful in accomplishing this is "hip hinging", which eliminates the spine as a source of motion and instead focuses such movement into the hips. We will learn more about hip hinging later.

2. Stand and rise up onto your toes. Drop down onto your heels – gently at first. This typically produces a compressive load of about one and a half times your body weight through your spine. Is pain or discomfort triggered? Record your findings. Repeat the heel drop, but this time, keep your neck flexed by bringing your chin to your chest. If you find that this flexed-neck drop stimulates pain, try the drop a third time with the flexed-neck in a position of extension. This can be reached by tilting the head back, in other words "looking up." If the pain is at its worst in a flexed position, but is alleviated in the extended position, then there is some neural component to your pain, which is modulated by neck posture. In other words, your body is indicating that a nerve is being pinched somewhere in your back. In looking up, you have found a posture that relieves tension in the nerve and provides pain relief. This doesn't mean that you have to live your life with your neck craned skyward. You have merely identified forward neck flexion as a trigger. Simple life hacks such as lowering your office chair to bring your eyes more level with your computer screen or chopping your vegetables on a higher surface than a standard countertop, will help you avoid this painful flexed position. Also stop stretching and avoid movements at the extreme ranges of joint motion to allow the nerve sensitivity to settle.

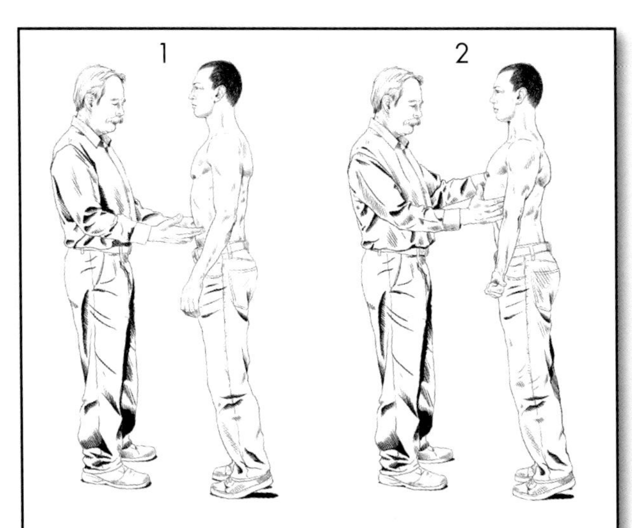

Test 2. The heel drop will determine if dynamic loads cause pain, and if the loads are influenced by posture and muscle stiffness (firmness). (1) Gently perform the heel drop without any muscular bracing – you are relaxed. Now repeat with stiffened and braced abdominal muscles. If pain is decreased you have found a pain relieving strategy for use in loading tasks. If the pain is increased then loading with abdominal bracing is not for you, at least not yet. (2) Now repeat the heel drop relaxing the abdominals but with stiffened and braced latissimus and pectoralis muscles, pulling the shoulders down into an anti-shrug position. Note if this strategy reduced pain.

What is the most painful muscle strategy?__________________

What is the least painful muscle strategy?__________________

If you had pain we will repeat the test and see if you can reduce the pain sensitivity. The goal is to put your neck into the posture that triggered pain but slightly stiffen or harden the abdominal muscles and repeat the drop. Is the pain gone, or reduced? If YES, then bracing and stiffening the core muscles will be a helpful tool in reducing your pain. You have found a muscular strategy to increase your resilience in activities that load the spine. Or is the pain worse? If YES, then you cannot tolerate the extra compression down your spine from abdominal bracing. Instead try shoulder bracing – pull and depress your shoulders down by contracting the pectoral and latissimus muscles. In other words, imagine your shoulders down and moving away from your ears. Repeat the drop, did the pain lessen? If so, you have found a muscular bracing pattern that allows you to increase your ability to handle loads pain-free.

Remember, by finding techniques to avoid your pain triggers, and experiencing longer periods of pain-free living, over time your pain will desensitize and you will be able to return to activities that once caused your back distress.

What reduced pain?__________________________

Abdominal bracing?__________________________

Pectoral and latissimus muscle bracing?______________

Postures that reduce pain:

The goal of these next tests is to help you discover which are your feel-good postures: the ones that will fast-track your recovery.

1. Leave this next test for when you are experiencing some pain. Stand and make a mental note of your level of pain. This will be your "baseline." Now lie on the floor on your tummy. Is this comfortable? If not, ease into it for approximately thirty seconds. If the pain persists or worsens, skip to the next test, this one is not for you. If this relieves pain, then maintain this position for 3 minutes. Then stand up without flexing the spine. The key is to push-up onto your hands and knees and lunge up, hinging through the hips instead of the spine. Once standing again is the pain now reduced? If so, the pain can be most likely traced back to a disc bulge. By lying in this position for three minutes, you have already slightly reduced the disc bulge and experienced some pain relief as a result. Regardless

of the source of your painful tissue, if this posture produces "feel-good" results, you have proven that flexion triggers your pain and that gentle, unloaded extension takes it away.

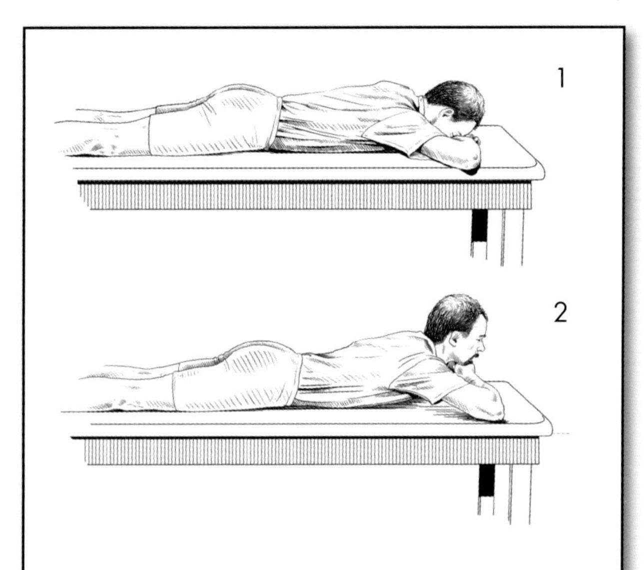

Test 3. Tummy lie. Lie on the floor for 3 minutes (stop after 30 seconds if pain is getting worse – but try and give it 30 seconds to see if it will settle). If position 1 is relieving try position 2 and compare if this is better or worse than 1. Stay with the more pain relieving version.

Does tummy lying reduce your pain when lying and when you return to standing?__________ (If so you have found a "go to" position when you need relief, or if you have "overdone" it).

If the above position in fact *causes* pain, then you may have pain triggered from extended postures. Let's work on finding a happy posture for you. To confirm, stand up and arch back through the lower back. Is this a pain aggravator? If yes, repeat the extension but with a twist to one side. Now try the other side. You may be able to discover that the extension plus rotation to one side causes your pain. If this is the case, stand on one leg (the same side as the pain). Stand tall as if you were beginning to march. Now repeat the pain causing extension. Is the pain less? If so you have proven that stiffening the pelvis and spine will make you more resilient to extension postures. For you a "feel-good" position is where the spine is neither flexed nor extended but in a neutral position.

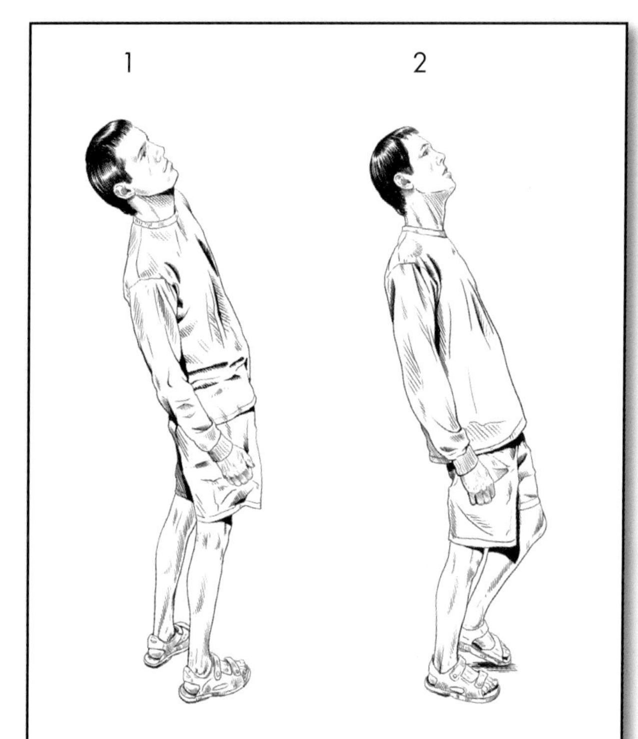

Test 4. Standing extension test. (1) First stand on both feet. Does extending and then twisting one way cause pain? (2) If YES stand on one foot – the same foot as the side of pain and repeat. Does this change the pain?

3. Next, plank on a wall by supporting yourself on your forearms. This creates a low-risk safe-zone to experiment with various postures. Slowly move through flexion and extension, first through your low back. Next experiment with flexion and extension through your hips. Ideally you will find a combined hip and spine posture that minimizes pain. Practice finding this pain reducing/eliminating posture starting from a neutral position. Ideally you will be able to incorporate this healthy posture in your daily activities. Try and modify activities like sitting in a car seat and walking the dog to more closely resemble the position found to be a pain-reliever.

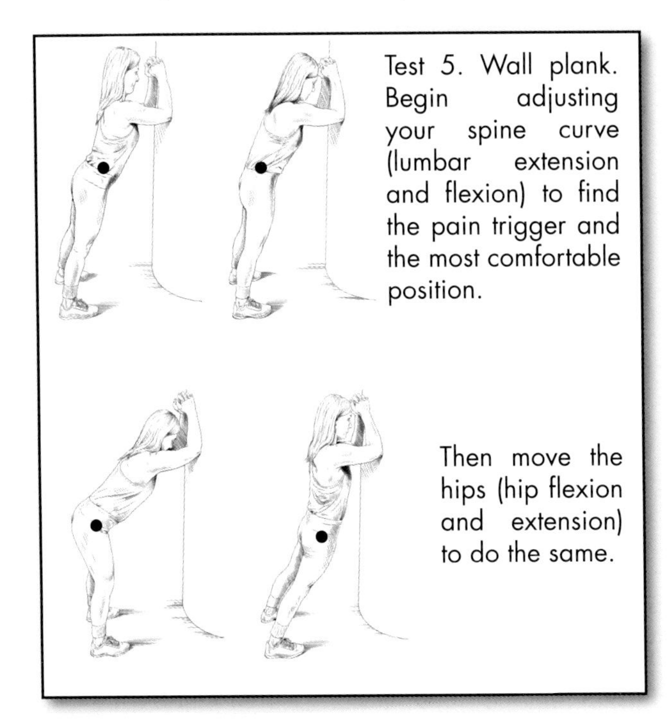

Test 5. Wall plank. Begin adjusting your spine curve (lumbar extension and flexion) to find the pain trigger and the most comfortable position.

Then move the hips (hip flexion and extension) to do the same.

Note the combination of hip and spine postures that minimize pain.____neutral____

Loads that cause pain:

This next exercise will identify whether the action of placing forces through your spine triggers your pain.

1. Take a five pound weight. Stand with your back in your pain-free posture. For most of you this should be neutral or a slight deviation from neutral. Hold it at your belt buckle. Observe and record any perceived pain. If you can perform this comfortably, then outstretch your arms holding the weight away from you. Is there pain this time? If YES, we can conclude that at your current stage, your back is very load intolerant. In terms of your daily life, this should translate into eliminating unnecessary loading of your back during your recovery. This means doing things like having someone help you unload heavy groceries and postponing activities like gardening until you are healthier. Here's a tool that can help you with minor loads in the meantime: adjust the abdominal muscles by stiffening your core and correcting any lax spine posture to see if pain can be eliminated.

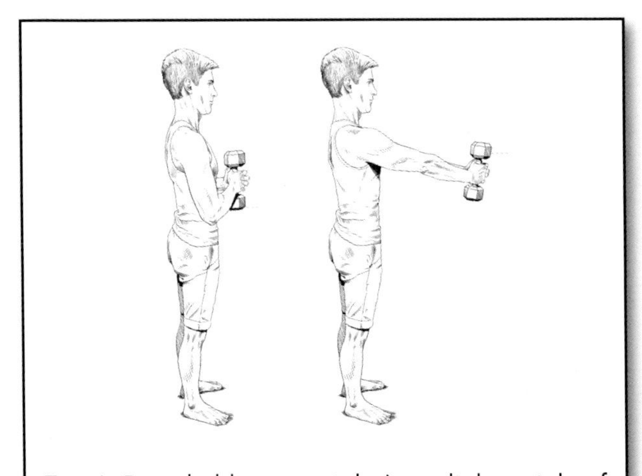

Test 6. Does holding a weight (try a light weight of 5 pounds (2kg)) increase pain? Be sure to adjust your spine curves to test whether a neutral spine curve reduces pain. Then try muscular bracing – does this reduce pain?

Does holding a load in front cause pain when your spine is in its pain-free postures?____no____

Can this be changed with muscular bracing?________

Motions that cause pain:

Let's look closely at a very common movement pattern that can be a pain trigger and examine how to eliminate it.

1. If you have already found your spine to be load intolerant, it is best to avoid this test. Place a bar or weight across your shoulders. Roll your pelvis bending the lumbar spine into flexion then into extension – excuse me but similar to the movement during sex. Does this motion cause pain? If so, lumbar motion is a trigger for you. It will be crucial to your recovery that you follow the instructions in the next section that will teach you to use your hips to bend rather than your spine. Many athletes have been successful in maintaining their ability to perform – you can too. Did moving in just one of the directions – either just flexion or just extension, cause pain? If so, note that you are intolerant of that motion and you will need to adapt your movement patterns to avoid the pain. The key to dealing with a motion intolerant spine is learning to stabilize your back and instead concentrate your movements in your body's major joints (ie. your shoulders and hips).

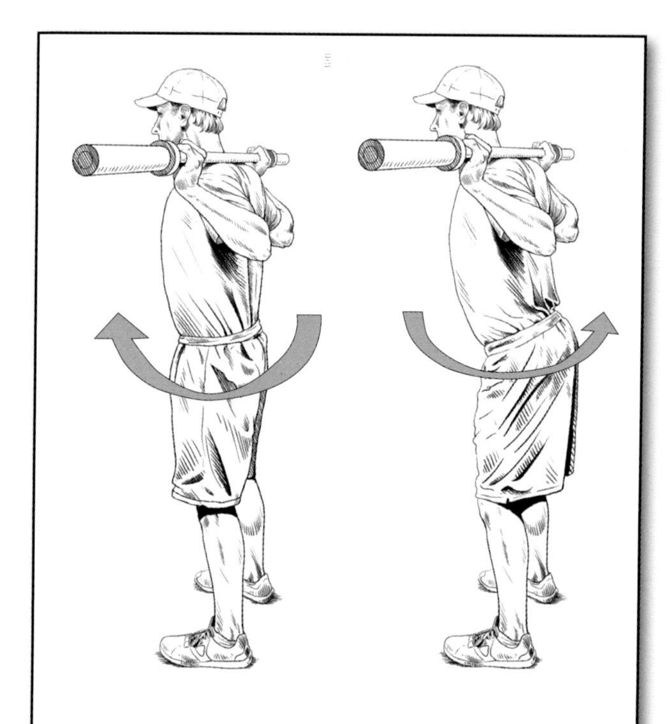

Test 7. The pelvic motion test for lumbar spine motion tolerance: Place a load on your shoulders – usually an unloaded bar will work well. Roll the pelvis, tilting forwards and backwards which causes lumbar spine motion. Does this trigger your symptoms or create discomfort?

Does flexion/extension movement increase your pain? _________

Assessment of posture and movement:

We have now covered the basics of a back assessment. You should have a few ideas from the first two sections of the self-assessment as to what is causing your pain. Let's follow this process a bit further.

1. Standing posture assessment. Standing tall without poking the chin or rounding-slouching the shoulders is ideal for reducing back load in most people. Here's a quick test. Poor posture causes these muscles to be on all day long. They are never given any relief. This causes muscular backache – now you know how to avoid it. Fix your standing posture. We will cover a stretch to help you correct this later. Here is a quick test.

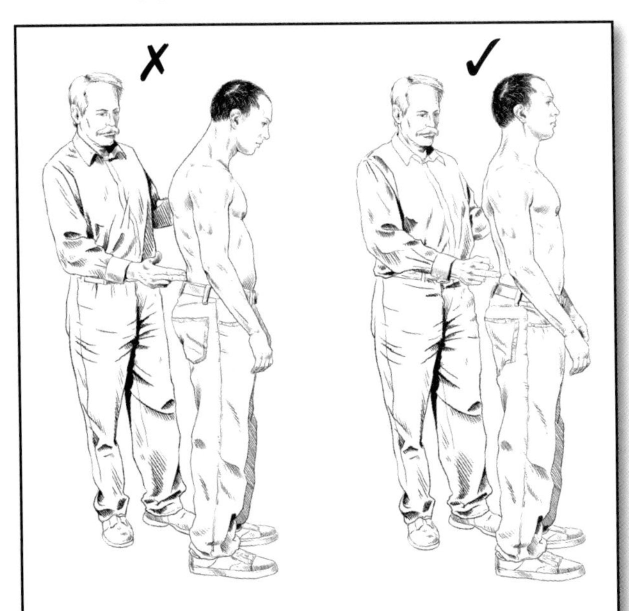

Test 8. Standing posture assessment. Find a standing posture to relax the low back muscles. Feel the low back muscles. Are they contracted and hard? If so, lean back into a more upright posture. You will feel the muscles relax. Examine what you needed to do to achieve this relaxed state. Now poke the chin – feel the muscles come on. Or round the shoulders into a slouched posture – again you will feel the back muscles come on. The idea is to stand and reduce the activity of these muscles. Failure to do so will cause muscle cramps.

What did you need to do to allow your low back muscles to relax?____

____

Typically in my assessments I will now assess movement patterns. These follow branching algorithms to really ferret out the movement flaws. Rather than take you through an extensive assessment that is needed for the most challenging patients, it is more prudent to simply show you ideal movement. This is in the next book section. Do not dismiss the importance of moving well.

To wrap up this section and gain true insight into your pain, you must pause and link the pain triggers you have identified, with movement patterns. When you brush your teeth, does it trigger pain? If so, is it because spine flexion triggers pain? Now you need to learn to brush your teeth without this trigger. Does reaching overhead trigger pain – is it because extension causes pain? What muscle stiffening strategy did you discover that reduced or eliminated the pain? As you work through the next section of the book, you will learn ways to move that avoid your pain triggers. Pay particular attention to positioning your spine in its pain-free and load resilient posture.

Note: If you feel that you have not been successful in identifying the triggers of your pain, see the section in a few pages that will guide a visit with a clinician to help you sort these out.

Step 4 – Assess your personality type as a recovery factor

We've already briefly discussed how personality type can affect back pain treatment success but it's worth discussing further. Here you must be honest with yourself. Does your personality tend more towards type A or type B? What's the difference? Type A's are hard-driving, making sure they accomplish everything on their to-do list today. Type A's push themselves and they push their backs. Typically, when I give a type A an exercise with eight repetitions as part of their routine, they will go away and do sixteen and then return wondering why their back didn't get better. They are ones who state they have to get to gym for their aerobics everyday, fearing that a day off will cost them their fitness. If this sounds like you, you *must* give yourself permission to take it easy. Recovery will not be possible if you continue to push yourself to your limits. Begin by removing what you have found to be your personal pain triggers, then *slowly* rebuild your tolerance for physical activity by mastering the rehabilitative exercises in the next section of the book.

In contrast, a type B individual with a more laid back personality will hear my prescription for eight reps and then think of an excuse as to why they only need to do four reps that day. If *this* scenario is more your style, it's time for you to step it up. If you're serious about ridding yourself of pain, you have to be serious about taking the steps needed to experience a proper recovery. Teach yourself to be more diligent with your daily regimen and you are more likely to succeed.

Both above examples are extremes, but both are equally problematic. Type A never gives their back a rest and remains in pain. Type B does not achieve the basic back fitness necessary to control postures and loads pain-free. If you're one of these extremes, you are encouraged to fight your natural tendency and find the middle ground.

Step 5 – Examining your pain category and recognizing patterns.

Each category of back pain is distinguishable by features. What helps one group may hurt another. Virtually all categories will be assisted with the "Big 3" exercises in their appropriate form, practicing appropriate spine hygiene principles, and interval walking which form the core program of this book. However, here are some general features with some specific guidelines for each category. Some of the recommendations have not been introduced yet – they will be in subsequent chapters.

Pain with spine flexion

Features: Pain is worsened with slouched sitting, bending and gardening or even tying your shoes.

Probable Cause: Almost always a disc bulge.

Pain relief: Lying on your tummy and allow your low back to fall to the floor with each exhalation.

Do this: Practice the "shortstop squat" and adapt it to all bending activities. Practice spine hygiene principles (all of these are coming in Chapter 8). Perform the Big 3 exercises.

Avoid this: When bending forward, avoid flexion motion in the spine and learn to "hip hinge." Avoid any single posture for a long time – for example sitting and standing.

Pain with dynamic loading

Features: Pain with walking up or down stairs, walking over uneven ground.

Probable Cause: Compressive injury to the vertebral end plate.

Pain relief: Lie on your tummy.

Do this: Practice abdominal bracing or pectoral-latissimus bracing and "tune" the brace to just reduce pain without over-bracing.

Avoid this: Avoid dynamic loading such as with running. Avoid exposure to vibration sources when sitting or standing such as with heavy equipment operation.

Pain with neck flexion

Features: Back, buttock or leg pain is increased with neck flexion which causes tension along the spinal cord.

Probable Cause: The nerve roots leaving the spinal cord have increased their sensitivity from mechanical irritation. Occasionally neck flexion relieves radiating pain – this usually indicates an "underhooked" nerve root from a disc bulge.

Pain relief: Find appropriate neck posture.

Do this: Begin with approaches to reduce the disc bulge such as tummy lying. Then consider nerve flossing after the corrective exercise program together with techniques of spine hygiene.

Avoid this: Do not stretch.

Pain with compression

Features: Pain with holding loads in front of you, or when opening a window for example.

Probable Cause: The cause could include compressive damage to the vertebrae or disc.

Pain relief: Experiment with spine hygiene principles.

Do this: Reduce the load with spine hygiene. Consider playing the "Virtual Surgery" recovery game.

Avoid this: Forward reaches.

Episodic back pain

Features: Periods of no pain interrupted with painful episodes that may vary from uncomfortable to excruciating.

Probable cause: Most likely the disc is the root of the pain. A flattened or bulged disc may press on a nerve, causing compression which often brings on radiating pains across the back, buttocks, groin and legs.

Pain relief: Certain postures can be found to relieve and conversely increase pain. Identify these. Avoid the painful ones.

> **KEEPING A LOG BOOK**
>
> Here is a method for sorting out the causes of your episodic pain – and what causes your painful days. Each day, record how your back feels. Also record the activities you perform, their duration, their intensity or applied load if relevant. Include the amount of rest, whether it be in a chair or lying down. Record the posture. Did you use a lumbar support while sitting? You get the idea. The more detail the better. Once you have four or five more painful days accumulated in the log, go back and review. You will find patterns. Specific patterns cause you to have a more painful day. Focus first on the day or two before the back pain flare-up. Was there an activity, or longer duration of activity that resulted in subsequent pain?

Do this: Identify the pain triggers and avoid them. You will need to recall what triggered the attack. Was it gardening, a sneeze, or sitting at work? You will need to avoid or modify the technique for the trigger.

Avoid this: The pain triggering postures.

Pain when walking a specific distance

Features: Initially walking is tolerable but soon becomes painful.

Probable cause: Usually associated with older people and arthritic conditions. If it occurs in younger individuals it is more likely a joint such as the sacroiliac joint or facet joint. Essentially cumulative loading of the disc and/or arthritic joints causes irritation of the local nerves and sometimes those travelling down the legs.

Pain relief: Find the pain relieving posture, usually sitting or lying. Avoid repetitive motions in the back.

Do this: Interval train "walking" into tolerable "chunks". Perform relieving postures following each "chunk". This will create tolerable walks and overall recovery over time.

Avoid this: Periods of walking long enough to stimulate the pain. Instead, end the walk while you're still feeling good.

Pain when bending backwards or when twisting

Features: Back pain triggered by bending backwards or twisting motions. Usually made worse when twisting is combined with spine extension. If the pain lessens when standing on one leg, there is instability associated with the pain.

Probable cause: Usually a combination of disc pathology with facet joint involvement.

Pain relief: Avoid spine extension and twisting.

Do this: Learn to move with the hips.

Avoid this: Avoid your pain-inducing postures and replace them with your "feel-good" ones.

It only hurts with specific exercises

Features: For example it only hurts when performing back squats or deadlifts.

Probable cause: Flawed mechanics overloading specific tissues or too much load or too high a training volume.

Pain relief: Avoid or modify the exercise.

Do this: Identify the pain trigger and movement flaw and remove them. Reduce the training volume. If you're dealing with weights, lower the amount you're dealing with and instead focus on healthy movement through pristine technique.

Avoid this: The motion found to be the pain trigger.

Step 6 – Dealing with Inconclusive Results

For the vast majority of cases, the above diagnostics will be very effective in revealing your personal pain triggers. Remember that naming your condition should come secondary to being able to identify what postures, loads and motions are the aggravators of your pain. The fact does remain that there is a small percentage of individuals that, after undergoing the above self-diagnostic tests, have varying results that do not point to any specific triggers. These individuals may have found that everything caused them the same level of pain, or that none of these provocative tests produced symptoms. Further still, there are the few cases that will receive mixed messages from their results that don't seem to point to an identifiable trigger.

This next suggestion works very well for individuals who have more painful and less painful days. The good news is they have the ability to have a good day. The bad news is they don't know how to create more of them. These people need to keep a log that will reveal their pain cause.

A very small number will fail to find patterns in their log book. For them, I would advise to seek out a reputable clinician and undergo further testing. Even some individuals who did find conclusive results may choose to get a second opinion (although I believe that if you've discovered the causes and relief mechanisms of your pain, you are armed with all the knowledge you need to continue to the next step alone). I urge you to acquire my textbook *"Low Back Disorders: Evidence-based Prevention and Rehabilitation"* which I wrote for the medical community. Take a copy to the clinician as a guide for them to conduct much more extensive tests on your hips, lumbar nerve roots, pelvic ring, sacroiliac joints, facet joints, etc. together with tests to reveal neural sensitivity, and muscle imbalance, to name a few. If you're a reader seeking to maximally expand your knowledge base, you are encouraged to read this book yourself. It also will act as a reference so that you are both "speaking the same language" as you proceed with your examination.

Seeking out the right caliber of professional advice will be challenging. And although the exam some clinicians will administer may not be comprehensive, you will be better armed to present them with the notes you took during your self-assessment. Don't be afraid to be your own best advocate for your back health.

Here are a few suggestions to assist you in making sure you get good advice.

Tests to be performed by your clinician

Through reading this book, you probably have a much better understanding of pain, pain triggers, and ways to avoid pain-inducing movements. I would hope that you also have an increased understanding of the physiology influencing your back and that you are also better equipped to ask specific questions of your practitioner regarding tests and results.

Testing: What constitutes a thorough examination?

Here is what the clinician with spine expertise should test and do. The medical professional needs to fine-tune, hone and further sub-divide categories of back pain. The elite medical professional gives direct guidance as to what you, the patient must stop doing and what you should do next. If a clinician fails to provide specific guidance as to the cause of your pain, and how to avoid it, you are not with a clinician competent with back pain and I would advise you to find an alternate. If all you receive is pain medication – you must find another clinician.

A clinician working towards a precise diagnosis will perform precise pain provocation tests. Think of the medic attending an injured athlete at a sports game. They begin by moving the body part in question (let's say the knee) through a variety of different motions and positions, asking the athlete "does this hurt?" The medic needs to deliberately incite pain in order to move forward in a diagnosis and to ultimately advise the athlete on how to heal and eliminate it. The same type of tests should be performed by a clinician using precise pain provocation tests.

The well-informed patient: Challenging, unresponsive back-pained patients deserve a competent assessment

One phrase back pain medical professionals often use is, "non-specific back pain." Sometimes they call it "Idiopathic back pain" or perhaps "Lumbosacral strain." When doctors and physiotherapists use such diagnostic terms what they really mean is "there is no diagnosis, there is no known cause of pain." I hope that by this point in the book you understand that all back pain can be traced back to a cause of some sort. We have been referring to these causes as triggers. One not-so-subtle inference made by branding someone's back pain as non-specific is that the pain is in the patient's head, nothing more than psycho imaginings. In its worst form the concept of non-specific pain is used by insurance companies to dismiss patients from their payrolls. Whatever your previous experiences, be assured that non-specific back pain is a myth. The following is what a competent clinician will review with you during a visit.

What every back-pained patient needs to know

While many of you will find this self-assessment sufficient, those requiring professional assessment should have specific expectations. The following components lead to an effective and thorough medical diagnosis, one that promotes and facilitates full, long-term recovery, together with a strategy to manage the symptoms over the short term. Here is what you should expect:

1. **Exam results:** Every patient deserves to be told (and have interpreted) their test results, scores and measurements. It is highly recommended that you take notes as the physician is speaking. If the doctor is using medical jargon that you don't understand, speak up! You should be able to walk away with enough of an understanding of your results that you could re-explain them to someone else in your own words.
2. **Natural history of your malady:** Every patient deserves to have their malady placed in a context. Like any condition, back pain has a natural medical history. While some tissue injuries, particularly those related to the disc, initiate a domino effect that results in longer lasting pain sensitivity, most can be effectively managed so pain is avoided. You should know what to expect going forward.
3. **A prognosis:** Every patient should be given a prognosis. In other words, a discussion should be had regarding the chances for a full and complete recovery over the long term, or at least the likelihoods of mastering the ability to obtain pain relief from their injury. Most back disorders can be managed so that pain is a rare occurrence while nature guides the spine through the healing process. When the injury has healed, and the spine has stiffened on its own, the patient will no longer experience pain at all.
4. **Prescription:** Not one to be filled by the pharmacist! Every patient should be prescribed posture and movement patterns that enable and maintain painless activity. Appropriate classifications of back pain and matched corrective treatments should be introduced. Specific remedial exercises should ideally be "tuned" as you check in with the clinician later on and continue to proceed down your rehabilitative path.
5. **Causes of pain:** Every patient deserves to have the cause of pain clearly determined and explained. A good clinician will show you the motions, postures and loads that cause immediate pain, together with delayed onset pain, then demonstrate alternative movements and postures that avoid these identified pain triggers.
6. **Recovery plan:** Every patient deserves to have a comprehensive plan outlined for them consisting of multi-dimensional corrective and therapeutic exercise progressions, with benchmarks to guide incremental steps. The initial progression focuses on the first objective (elimination of pain). Once this goal is successful, the second objective is to expand activity range and enhance pain-free performance. Essentially, you want your recovery plan to be able to grow with you as your pain is reduced. Start small and dream big!

Assessing Assessments

After having met with a clinician, review the session in your mind as well as in the notes you have taken. Have you been given the assessment you deserve? Here are some thoughts to consider:

- Only a few very skilled clinicians will be able to diagnose back troubles based on anatomical structure. What happens if there is more than one pain-generating tissue? Only a surgeon who is attempting to "cut the pain out" will be looking to precisely identify which tissue is the primary pain source. Sadly, some fail to correctly pinpoint the problem area and operate on the wrong tissue. If you are with the surgeon, ensure that they are certain of the pain source. Otherwise, the session should have been focused more on controlling the motions, postures and loads that trigger pain rather than the actual tissues themselves.
- Back pain is almost always made worse by one particular motion, posture or load that the back-pained patient habitually repeats over and over. You should come away from the assessment with an understanding of what your personal triggers are and where in your daily life you are most likely to experience them. This knowledge paired with avoidance strategies are the keys to recovery.
- Your prevention plan should be designed to eliminate specific painful motions, postures and loads identified through provocative testing.
- The rehabilitation plan should be designed to enhance pain tolerance and teach alternative movement patterns.
- Back-pained patients should be subcategorized, based on their respective pain intolerances. Examples of categories include: episodic back pain, pain when walking a specific distance, pain when bending backward or when twisting, and probable cause.
- The proper assessment doesn't use a catch-all phrase such as "degenerative disc disease." There is no such thing.
- The proper assessment provides clear clinical direction with an alternate plan in case the proposed approach does not achieve the expected results within a given timeframe.

For the most challenging patients: Diagnosis by hypothesis testing

Occasionally some pains are difficult to detect and understand. To make matters more complicated, there may be more than one cause of the painful disorder. The more complex patients will require an expert diagnostician. These are the difficult patients I see.

A diagnosis by hypothesis testing will be helpful to sort out complex patients who do not produce conclusive signs during simple assessments. Once the assessment has arrived at a conclusion, the rehabilitation program becomes "an experiment in progress". Here, only one variable in a rehabilitative program is altered at a time. A daily diary records these to help me link the treatment plan with the progress. Thus, if improvement is made, or if the pain becomes worse, the offending variable can be isolated. This is a longer process, but the approach helps me to sort out the most complex patients.

In Summary

Through the right self-assessment, most people will be able to identify the postures, loads and motions that are their personal triggers for back pain. They should also be able to distinguish if neural tension is a factor contributing to their issues. Remember that during recovery, what you *don't* do is often just as important as what you *do* do. Cut out the aggravating actions and replace them with healthy ones. Most of your daily activities can be modified to better suit you.

When dealing with a physician-administered exam, remember the following: the Master Clinician "teaches" the patient the cause of their pain. If your clinician has not shown you the specific cause of your pain, then you need to consider engaging the services of another clinician.

Section 3:
The Repair Job: Making activity pain-free

Recall the 80% club – members following this program will get better. The remaining 20% will also begin here but will need some special modifications that follow in the next section of this book. Let's cover the general plan now.

1. Eliminate the cause of the pain and find pain free postures (lying, sitting, standing)
2. Develop posture and movement patterns that enable you to function pain-free
3. Essential exercises for everyone to stabilize the torso, core and spine when moving through life (the Big 3)
4. Develop a walking plan
5. Mobilize the hips
6. Make daily use of exercises based on patterns of movement: push, pull, carry, etc.
7. Make healthy spine choices when engaging in any activity

Chapter 7

Removing the Cause of Pain: Learning Basic Movement Tools

Removing the Cause of Pain

Learning Basic Movement Tools

From reading the previous chapters you should have a good idea at this point of which postures and movements create and exacerbate your pain. You have also become aware of those postures and movements that relieved pain. Here we follow a step-by-step guide to incorporate pain-free movements into your daily life.

For the chronic back-pain sufferer, winding down pain sensitivity requires you to move in the most spine-conserving way possible. For those with repeated acute pain attacks, this is the key to their avoidance in the future. Our pain-free posture and movement strategies must be rooted in being mentally aware and engaged. Your success rests in your ability to move mindfully and to avoid mental lapses and periods of inattention. Be conscious and aware of your movement. If you can maintain a lasting sense of spine-sparing body awareness, pain-free movement will soon become automatic.

The following exercises might at first glance seem simple, but I urge you to pay attention to the details as you execute them.

Let's begin by mastering the abdominal brace. This should be your basic building block: the technique you maintain as you continue to learn additional movement patterns.

The Abdominal Brace

Recall that core stiffness is required in order to prevent painful spine joint micro-movements and to allow more movement in the hips and shoulders. This is achieved through the abdominal brace, an important tool in your back health toolkit. The abdominal brace is a different concept than that of simply holding in your stomach. "Sucking in your stomach" or "pulling your navel to your spine" have both been lauded as healthy bracing techniques for the spine. This idea, however, is another harmful back myth popularized by some schools of Physical Therapy, Pilates and various other fitness trends.

True bracing is a mild contraction of the abdominal muscles as though you are preparing to be punched in the mid-section – but contract mildly. Now "tune" the brace to the task. When I say tune, I'm asking you to gradually adjust the amount of the contraction to find the optimal stiffness, much like a dimmer switch gradually adjusts light levels in a room. In the same way, you want to avoid going from one extreme to the other in the way an ON/OFF switch would function. Add more bracing stiffness for lifting heavy objects and apply less bracing for activities where spine posture control is needed, like when walking, or for rising from a chair. Exert just enough bracing stiffness to remove your pain and no more.

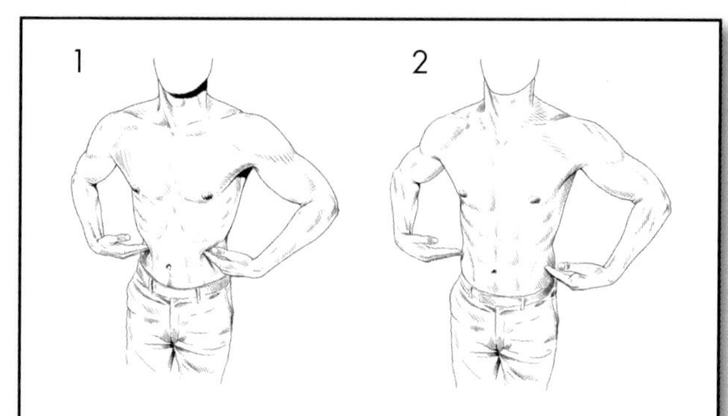

The abdominal brace: (1) with your abdominal muscles relaxed, push your fingers into the oblique muscles about 5 to 12 cm lateral of the navel. These are lateral to the rectus abdominis. (2) Do not suck the muscles in, rather gently stiffen the abdominal wall feeling the fingers being pushed out. Do not suck the muscles in, nor push them out. Simply activate them.

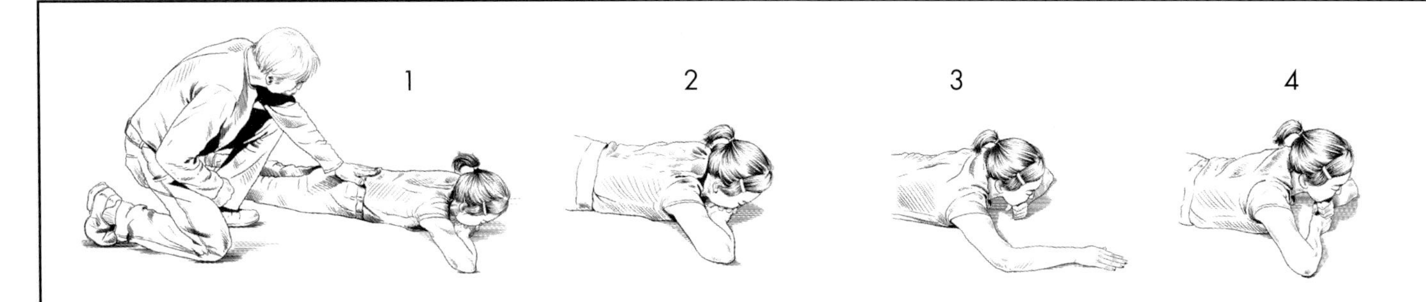

Lie face down and relax (1, 2). With each breath focus your thinking on your low back – allowing it to relax into the floor with each exhalation. If this is a relieving posture then make a fist under your chin (3). Then make two fists stacked one upon the other under your chin (4). If this is uncomfortable, go back to one fist. Lie like this for 3 minutes.

Finding Pain Free Postures (lying, sitting, standing)

If you are in acute pain at the moment, more exercise will not help. The first task is to reduce your pain. Pain often produces an "antalgia," meaning a loss of the normal spine "hollow." This antalgia leads to the unnatural flattening of the low back. Our goal is to restore the natural curve to the lumbar spine. Let's begin by experimenting with the following drill.

Lying down

Lie down on your stomach, with your hands flat under your chin. This should prop your head up so that you are looking forward. Take 20 seconds in this position. If you find that your pain has not increased, continue. Now place a vertical fist underneath your chin: little finger of the fist sits on the floor and your thumb and forefinger circle and cradle your chin. Is this better or worse in terms of pain? If it's better, try relaxing the face and neck muscles and sinking into this posture. Continue to breathe and relax deeper and deeper. Let the low back area sink to the floor with each exhalation. Focus your breath into restoring the natural hollow into your low back. If the fist makes the pain worse, regress back to having a flat hand under your chin, or even nothing under your chin and lay your head on its side. If this still increases pain then stop the lying posture.

If this is relaxing, comfortable and pain-free, try stacking a *second* fist atop the first. Now you have your chin resting on two vertical fists, stacked one atop the other, while lying on the floor on your stomach (see figure). Again, with this two-fist posture, seek to relax and breathe deeply into your lower back. For some, this may produce a slight feeling of stretching. The relaxed bow in your low back is both therapeutic and beneficial. If this double-fist version helps, add it to your postural repertoire until the daily pain reduces. If it is uncomfortable, withdraw back to just a single fist. You have now found another helpful pain-free posture!

Now stand up, trying to not move your spine as you stand. Use the same technique employed in the self-examination section. We will also break down this technique further in the following pages.

Now you are standing erect. Do you feel better or worse following the lying session? Has your sciatica or leg numbness disappeared? If you feel better, then congratulations! You have discovered another alternative pain-avoidance motion pattern, one that eliminates spinal flexion. Try lying on your stomach and repeating this fist under chin/stand-up sequence every few hours. Really focus on relaxing the muscles of the neck and back into this position. Stay quiet and remain in this posture for upwards of three minutes. Remember that you're trying to restore lordosis (or the lower back's natural hollow). Oftentimes, even a simple drill such as this allows the patient to overcome acute pain associated with everyday repetitive movements. For those who are made worse with this drill, we move on to another approach.

Sitting

Let's now focus our efforts on finding a low stress method of sitting that aids in pain relief. Sit in an office chair where you can see yourself in a mirror (see pic). Allow yourself to sink into a slouched position. Then sit up. Note if your movement strategy between the two positions was to lift the chest or if it was to roll the pelvis forward (see pic). The preferred movement pattern to achieve a relaxed spine without imposing muscular stress is to do a bit of both - roll the pelvis and lift the chest. Master this corrective movement to achieve a sitting posture with less stress and pain.

You will probably benefit from a lumbar pad (we prefer the Lumbair, www.backfitpro.com) to maintain this stress-free sitting posture (see pic – page 79). Use this corrective sitting when watching TV and working on the computer etc. But note, this cannot be achieved sitting on a soft couch. Your spine depends on a firm surface when sitting for proper support. It is also worth noting that although getting "comfortably" curled up on the couch with pillows that bring your head forward or slouching into an unsupportive surface like a bean-bag chair may feel good at first, in the long run you are not doing yourself any favours. This "feel-good" sensation is triggered by the same stretch reflex that occurs when you bring your knees to your chest while on your back. In both cases, this sensation of relief is fleeting, as you are actually placing added strain on your discs. You must avoid this posture.

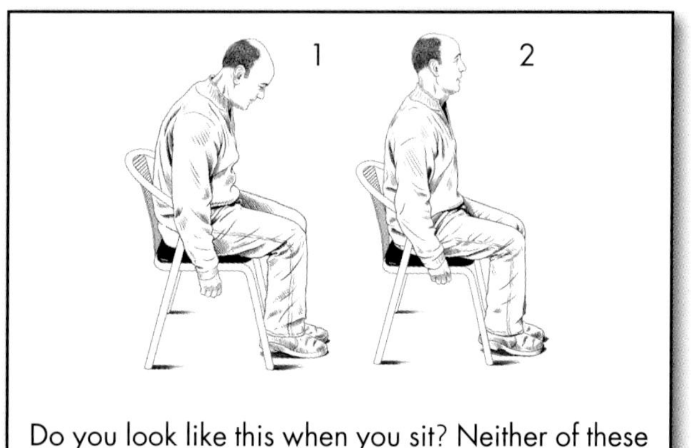

Do you look like this when you sit? Neither of these results in the lowest spine stress. The slouched spine is stressed (1) while the low back remains stressed (2) as it is not supported.

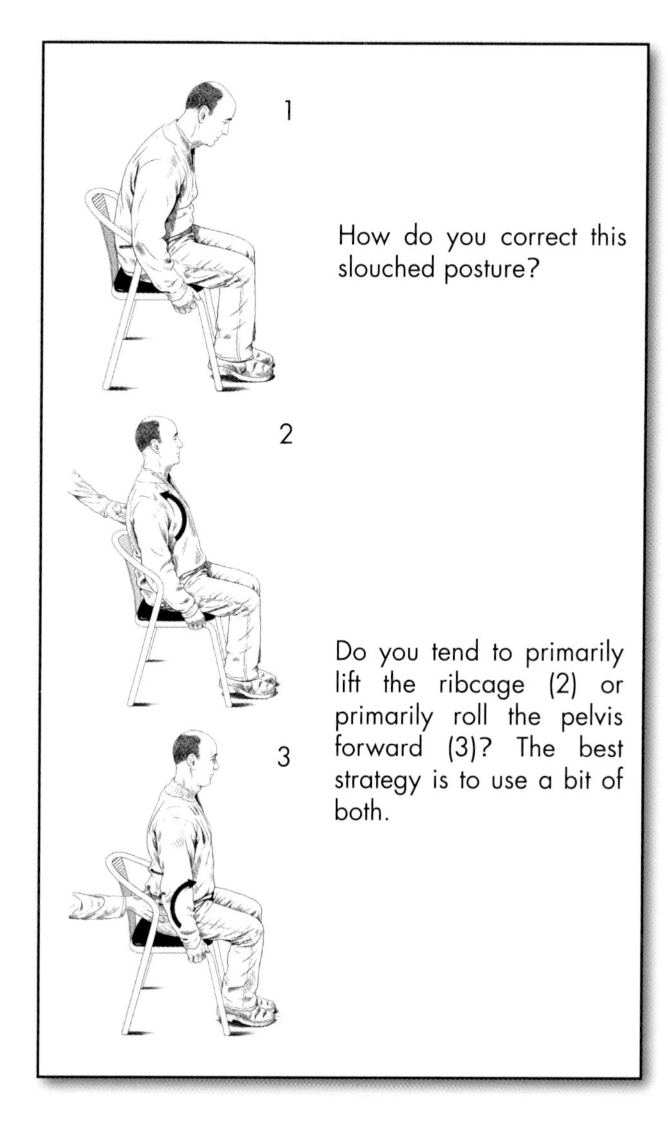

How do you correct this slouched posture?

Do you tend to primarily lift the ribcage (2) or primarily roll the pelvis forward (3)? The best strategy is to use a bit of both.

Use a lumbar pad (Lumbair) to eliminate lumbar spine stress when sitting. "Tune" the curve of the spine by adjusting the inflation level of the pad with the hand pump.

Standing

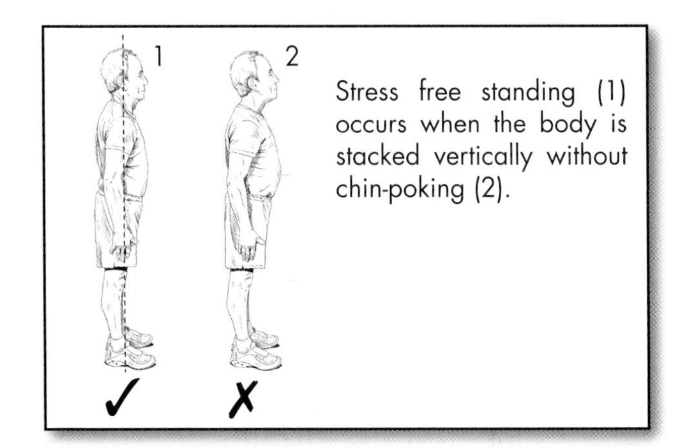

Stress free standing (1) occurs when the body is stacked vertically without chin-poking (2).

When standing upright and motionless, do you experience back stress? Feel the low back muscles with one hand (or have a friend do it for you) when standing. Are these muscles active and hard or relaxed and soft? The goal is to stand with relaxed muscles. Now here is how to find that position.

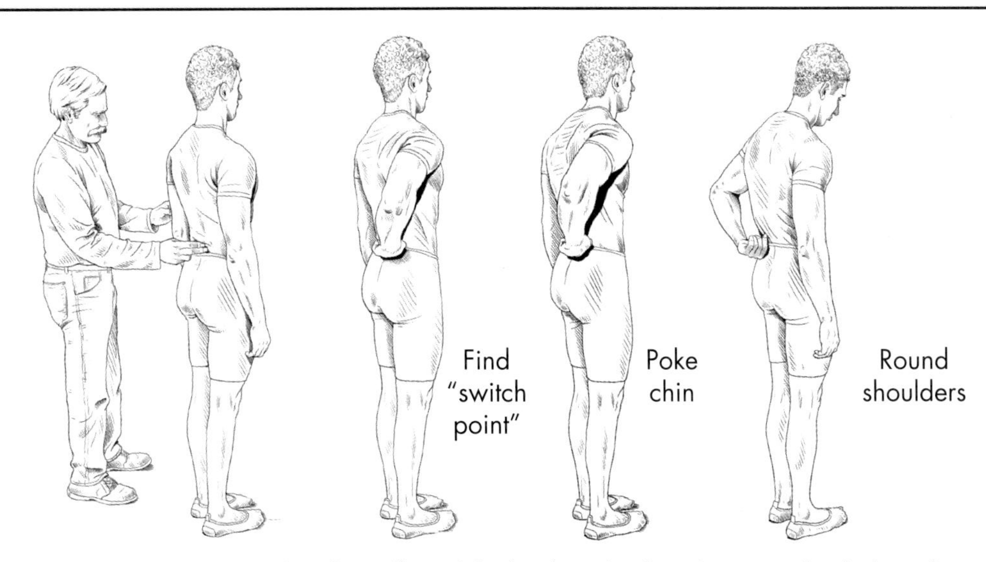

Try this drill: Lean slightly back until the muscles shut off (and feel soft and relaxed). Now slowly lean forward until you identify the point at which they become active and hard again. It may take a few passes to detect this muscle "switch point" but it is worth it. The objective is to discover the position that allows you to maintain an upright standing posture, without engaging your back muscles. Rounding shoulders and chin poking cause unwanted muscle tension. You see how important standing posture is to relax your back muscles.

Several postural features influence this stress free posture. Learn to control your pain while reducing stress and pain with this drill. Now that you've provided a self-demonstration on how these factors affect standing posture, use them to your advantage. Continue to remain aware of them when giving yourself a postural adjustment with the intent of relaxing your back muscles and you will experience greater success with alleviating your own pain.

Use this drill to gain skill in reducing standing stress: return to the position that "shuts off" your pain. While still feeling the relaxed muscles (1), poke your chin forward (2). You should feel your back muscles activate. Proceed to draw in the chin and feel the muscles relax. Next, try rounding your shoulders. You will feel the muscles contract. Moving your shoulders back to their upright position will relax the muscles. Holding the arms across the chest causes muscle cramps (3). Relieve the cramps by positioning the hands behind the back to shut off the low back muscles (4).

Another often neglected component when achieving a healthy standing posture is the position of the arms. Many of us, when standing in a "relaxed" upright position will cross our arms. This position encourages the rounding of the shoulders, and in turn the engaging of the back. Try instead, to keep your arms at your side, or even try clasping your hands behind your back. This will naturally and gently open your chest, relaxing the muscles in your back.

Also consider returning to the wall plank drill from the previous chapter. This will assist you in perfecting a strategy to reduce pain by altering your low back curve and hip posture. Next time you have pain when standing or walking, pause and try this technique.

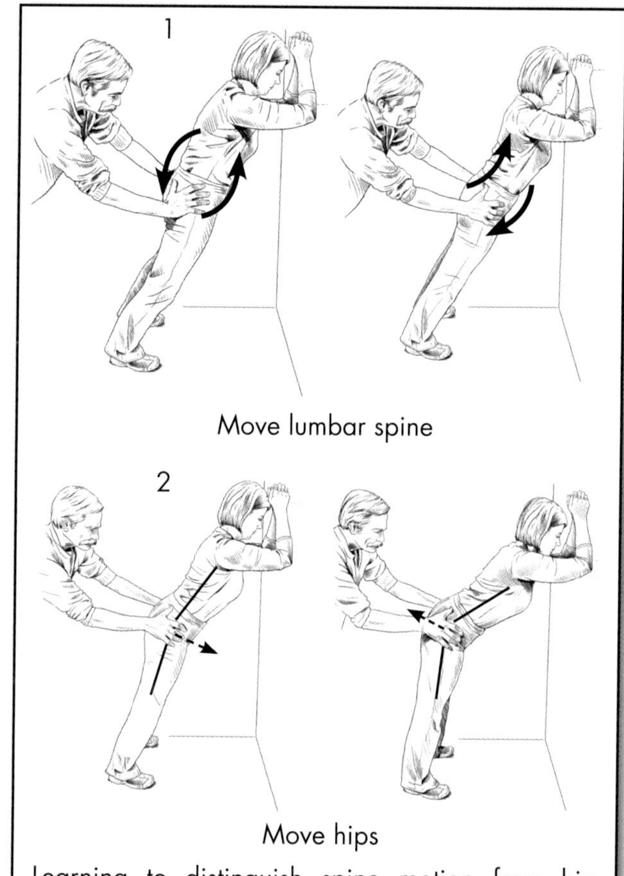

Learning to distinguish spine motion from hip motion. Flex and extend the lumbar spine to find the "sweet spot" of no pain (1). It helps to have this coached by a skilled clinician. Then work the pelvis to the wall with hip motion (2). This strategy will help you find the pain-free posture when out performing a daily activity such as shopping.

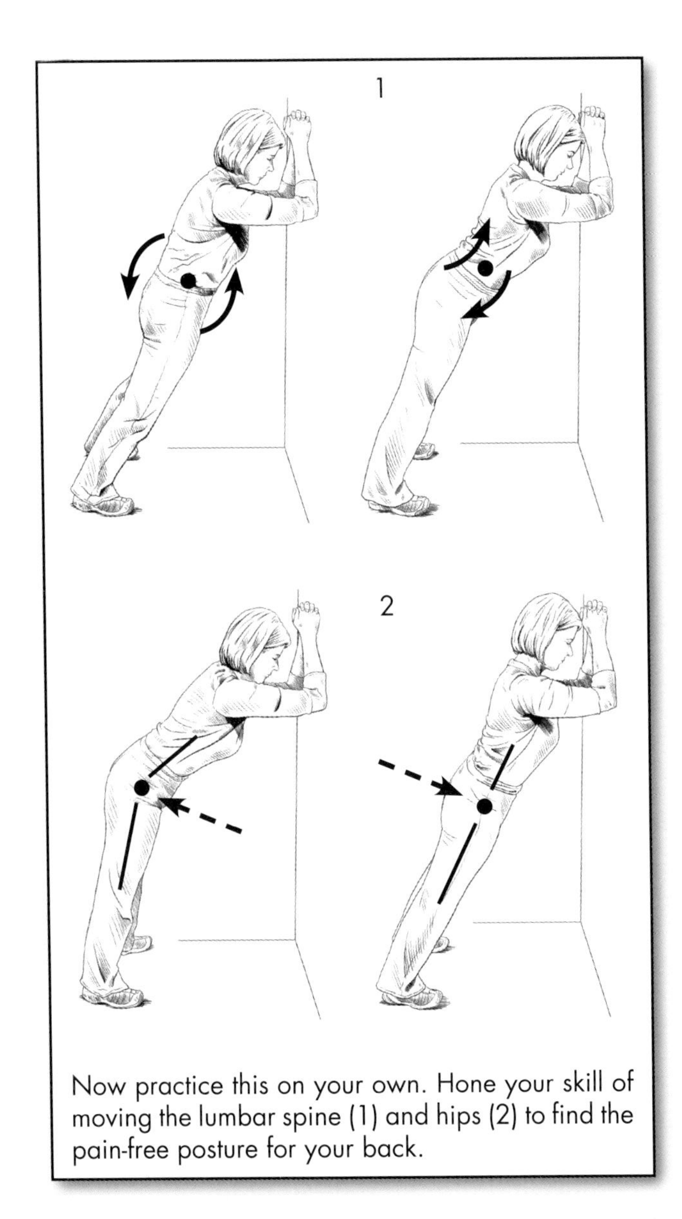

Now practice this on your own. Hone your skill of moving the lumbar spine (1) and hips (2) to find the pain-free posture for your back.

The Three Pain-Free Movement Tools

There are three basic movement patterns that must be mastered to develop a repertoire of pain-free movement. In fact, nearly all of life's chores can be accomplished in a spine sparing way by adopting these movement tools. The squat tool (1) can be used as a transition into sitting or to pick up an object that does not need you to place your hands to the floor. The lunge tool (2) is a movement pattern that is used to obtain a lying position on the floor, and rise up again to a standing posture with no pain. The stop twist tool (3) stops motion in the painful low back when performing tasks such as opening and closing doors. Master these, then develop the discipline to correctly choose one or more of the three when accomplishing a daily task pain-free.

1. The squat

The squat style developed here may be described as a hip-hinge. Proper squatting technique is not as easy to master as it might seem at first glance so be sure to pay attention to the details. This will be your basic tool for lifting everything from groceries to kids, or rising from the kitchen, office or movie theater chair, all pain-free.

The shortstop squat

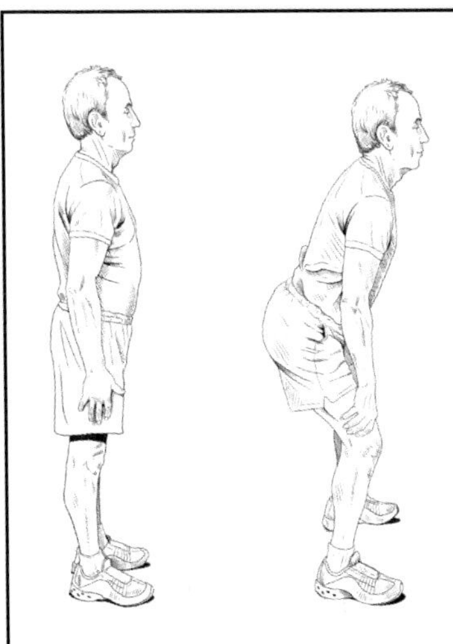

Here is a procedure I use to help beginners learn proper squat technique: Begin by standing erect with your feet spread shoulder width apart. Place your hands on your thighs. The space between the maximally opened forefinger and thumb form a "crotch." Keeping your spine straight, and bending at the hips, slide your hands down your thighs, directing your pelvis back behind you until you have lowered yourself to a point where the finger/thumb-crotch of each hand can be placed atop and around the kneecap. At this juncture your posture resembles the crouched postural position of a baseball shortstop.

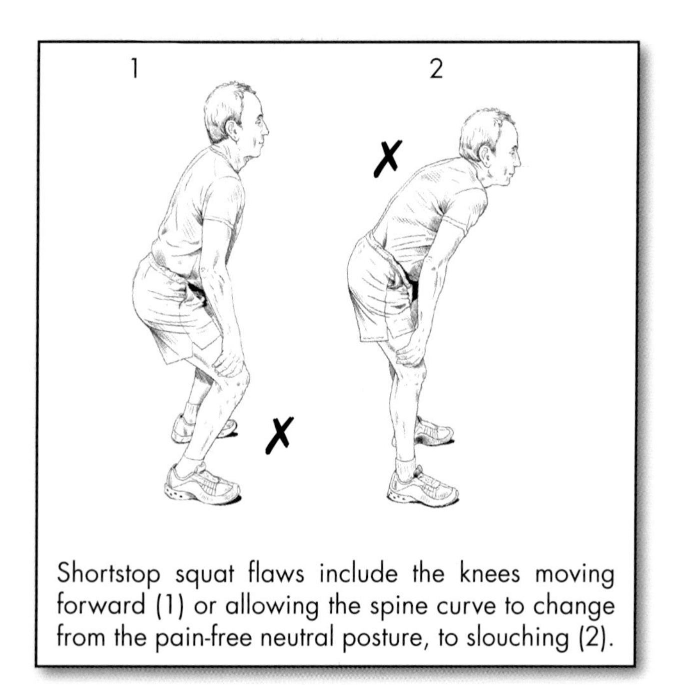

Shortstop squat flaws include the knees moving forward (1) or allowing the spine curve to change from the pain-free neutral posture, to slouching (2).

Work at finding and maintaining the pain-free spine curves or "sweet spot posture". Learn to stiffen the back, depressing the shoulders by activating the latissimus and pectoral muscles and carry the weight of your torso down the arms to the knees.

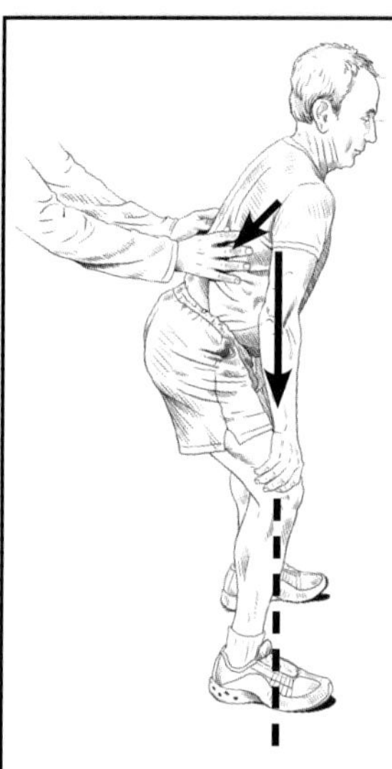

When you descend to the lowest squat position, the knees should fall in line mid-way between the heels and toes. Keeping the hands on the knees, adjust the knees to ensure this posture. Now it is time to move from this position into standing erect. Begin by stiffening the torso by invoking the "abdominal brace" – just enough and not too much. Now, instead of thinking of a shrug, do the opposite – anti-shrug. Picture pushing your shoulders down, away from your ears. Pushing down through the shoulders using the pectoral and latissimus muscles will allow your stiff arms to transmit weight to the knees. Feel your body weight being carried down your arms. Continue to maintain the hollow in your low back or slightly tune this posture to make it pain-free. This means slightly adjusting the lumbar curve to eliminate pain, but always aiming to work the spine towards a "neutral posture". The image of "lifting your tail" helps some. Now you must think differently in order to unload your back. Instead of *lifting* with your back, simply stiffen the supporting muscles. Focus on the abdominal brace and the stiffening of the latissimus and pectoral muscles as you protract/depress the shoulders downwards. Now concentrate on "pulling your hips forward", while maintaining a stiff back, as you draw your hands up the thighs. Motion should only occur at the hips. Continue this forward pelvic motion until you are standing back upright.

In summary, your mental focus should be on moving the hips back while descending into the squat and on pulling your hips forward while ascending into a standing position.

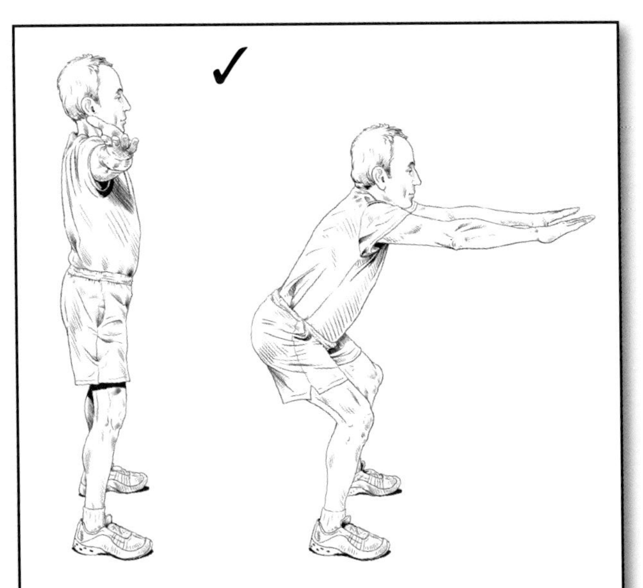

The arm assisted squat is used to train the squat pattern. Begin with the hands supinated (palms up). As the squat progresses the arms are brought forward to assist in balancing the body and the hands are pronated (palms down). Notice the hips flex to take the pelvis back (imagine sitting back, not down). The knees remain over the feet (half-way between the toes and heel).

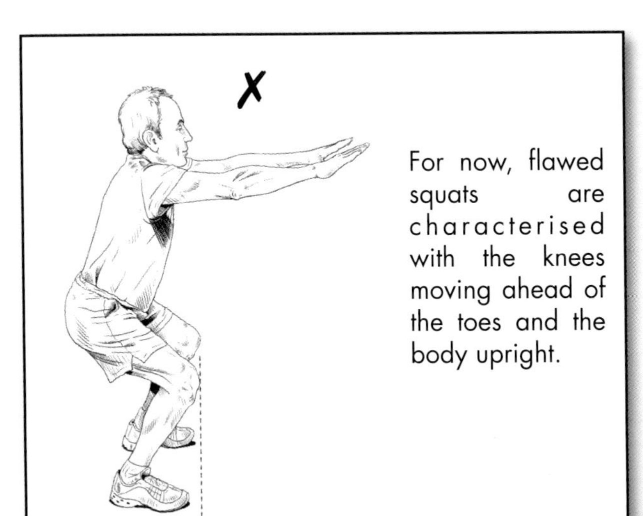

For now, flawed squats are characterised with the knees moving ahead of the toes and the body upright.

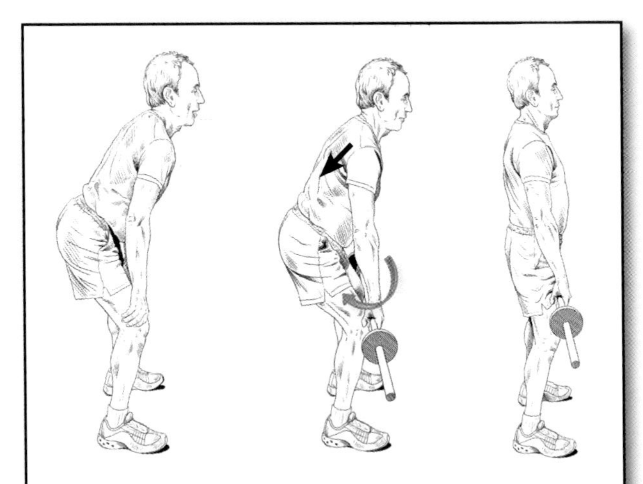

Now try lifting a bar. Grab a bar and adopt the shortstop position. "Twist" the bar with latissimus dorsi to stiffen the back. Then, do not lift with the back, rather, focus attention to simply pull the hips forward and drag the weight up the thighs.

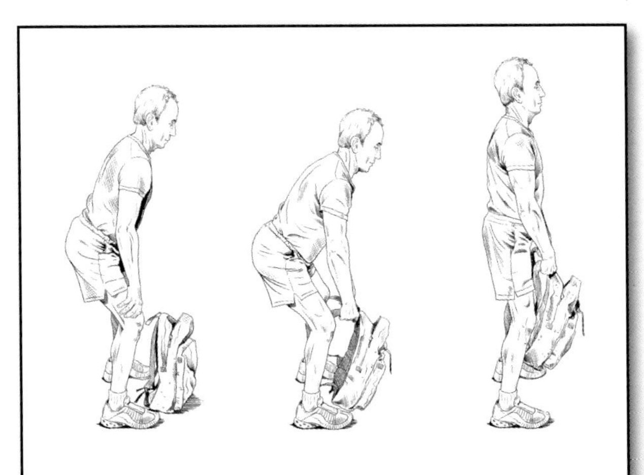

"Practice-lift" other objects with this pattern. Lock and stiffen the back and drag the object up the thighs by pulling the hips forward. The lift to upright will be pain-free.

The trick is to practice enough that this becomes a default pattern of moving when bending over to pick up an object or bending down to pat the dog. Over time, we will extend the range of motion, and continue to squat a little deeper with each repetition. For now, the complete squat novice should simply start off by practicing the basic pattern throughout the day. As the squat becomes more natural and habitual, you will find that your back, leg and hip strength has increased. The result is an improved ability to negotiate stairs, chairs, beds, showers, as well as an increased sense of ease when walking and getting in and out of a vehicle.

You will recall that incorporating the shortstop squat into daily activities was a significant part of spine hygiene.

The Chair Squat

Resist the urge to progress to other forms of the squat too soon. Once you feel as though you've mastered the shortstop squat technique, a variation of the exercise may be progressed.

One helpful practice is to stand in front of a standard height chair and sit back (move the hips rearward) improving your squat technique as you move into the chair. Focus on maintaining muscular tension and control even after your pelvis first makes contact with the seat of the chair. At no point should you give into the temptation to collapse back, using the chair to cushion you. To complete the drill, stand by pulling the hips forward. As you continue to perfect your form, remember to channel the movement of your squat down and back, as opposed to simply bending over and folding yourself in half.

One common lapse in form as people attempt this manoeuvre, is that their stance is too narrow to provide a proper base. Be sure to keep your feet wide enough apart (for most people, slightly wider than shoulder width should suffice). Be sure to maintain your wide foot stance during your ascent from the chair as well, however this time you will want to set up the squat by pulling them slightly underneath yourself. Then, instead of bending forward about the spine, initiate the upward movement by lifting the rib cage and bending the torso forward about the hip, all the while keeping your arms outstretched. While in this position, a sharp nasal inhale "sniff" will add beneficial stiffness to your spine. As you begin to stand, transfer the weight onto your feet and utilize the squat mechanics learned to rise into a fully erect stance. Practice this "chair squat".

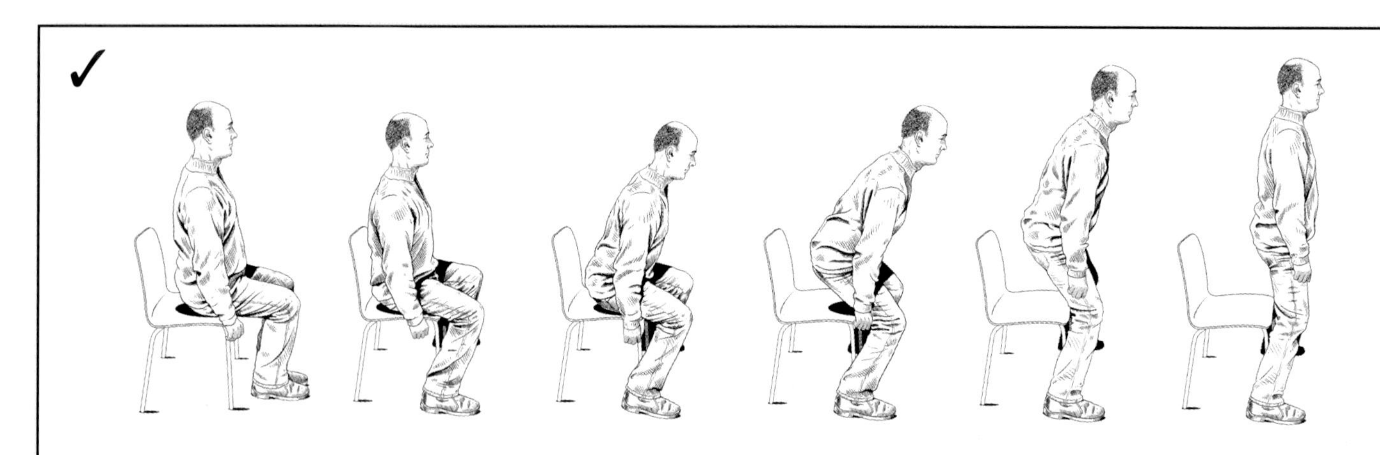

Rising from the chair in a spine sparing way. First spread the knees and position the feet underneath you. Lift the chest and lean forward through the hips, not through spine bending. Transfer the weight onto the middle of the feet with the pelvis still "back". Now move to upright by thinking about "pulling the hips forward", not lifting with the back.

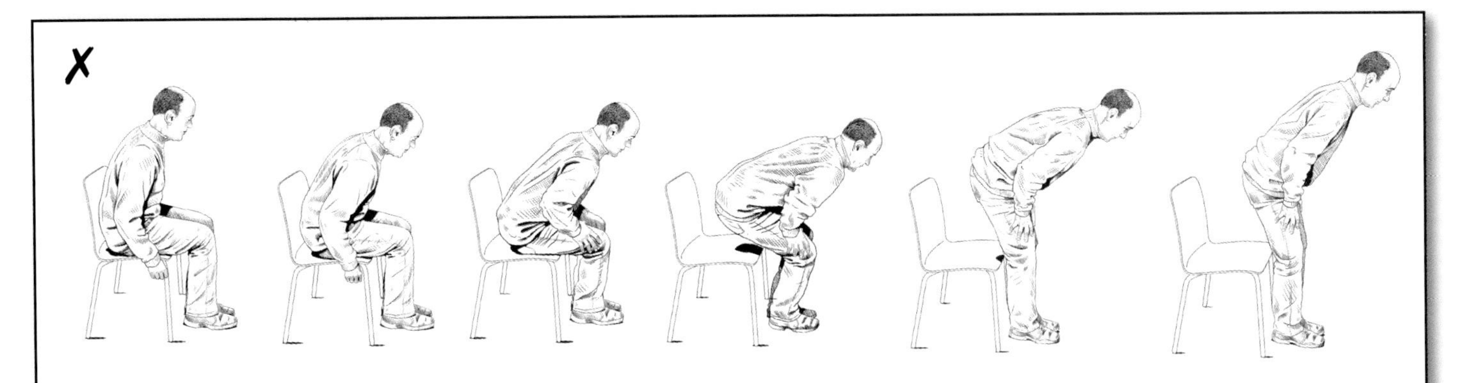

Poor form to rise from a chair leads to pain. Here the knees remain together and the feet remain in front of the person. The upper body is bent through the spine to posture the weight over the feet. The torso weight is then lifted with the back while in a flexed posture – guaranteeing pain.

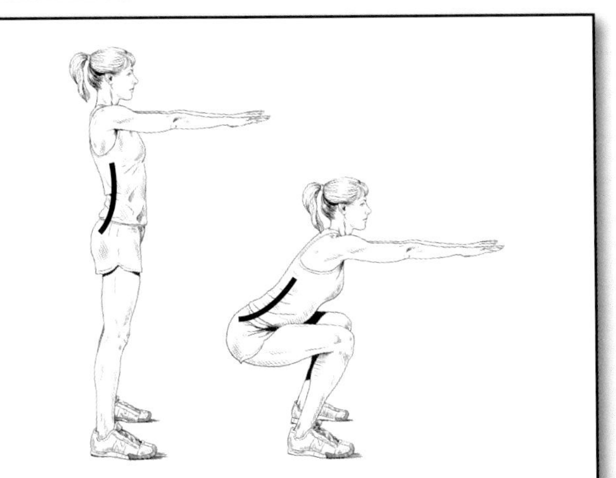

When you feel comfortable with this exercise, move on to the next phase. This time, as you squat back into the chair, you no longer need to slide your hands down your thighs for support. Instead, keep your arms outstretched straight in front of you and use them as a counterbalance as you move down and back. Do not squat deeply enough to allow loss of the neutral spine curve.

Pain-free squatting is a technique that can be employed to aid in a multitude of day-to-day tasks. Essentially every time you sit, stand, reach for something low or "duck down" you are performing a variation of a squat. Practicing proper technique will ensure that you are able to complete any of these tasks without placing added strain on your spine.

2. *The Lunge*

The lunge is the movement tool used to transition from a standing posture to lying down– this ability is important when getting in position to perform your floor exercises. Many people find this task impossible without pain until they master this spine-sparing lunge. Pay close attention to the pictures as you follow the step-by-step guide to achieving the perfect lunge.

Begin by finding your predetermined "sweet spot" of spine posture that is pain-free, then stiffen the core muscles so that no spine motion occurs. Try marching while maintaining this muscular control to ensure that all motion is only about the hips and not the spine (see walking chapter). Regulate spine motion so that no pain is triggered during any phase. Now that you've laid the ground work, let's begin.

Use this movement tool to get out of bed, up off the floor, even tie your shoes.

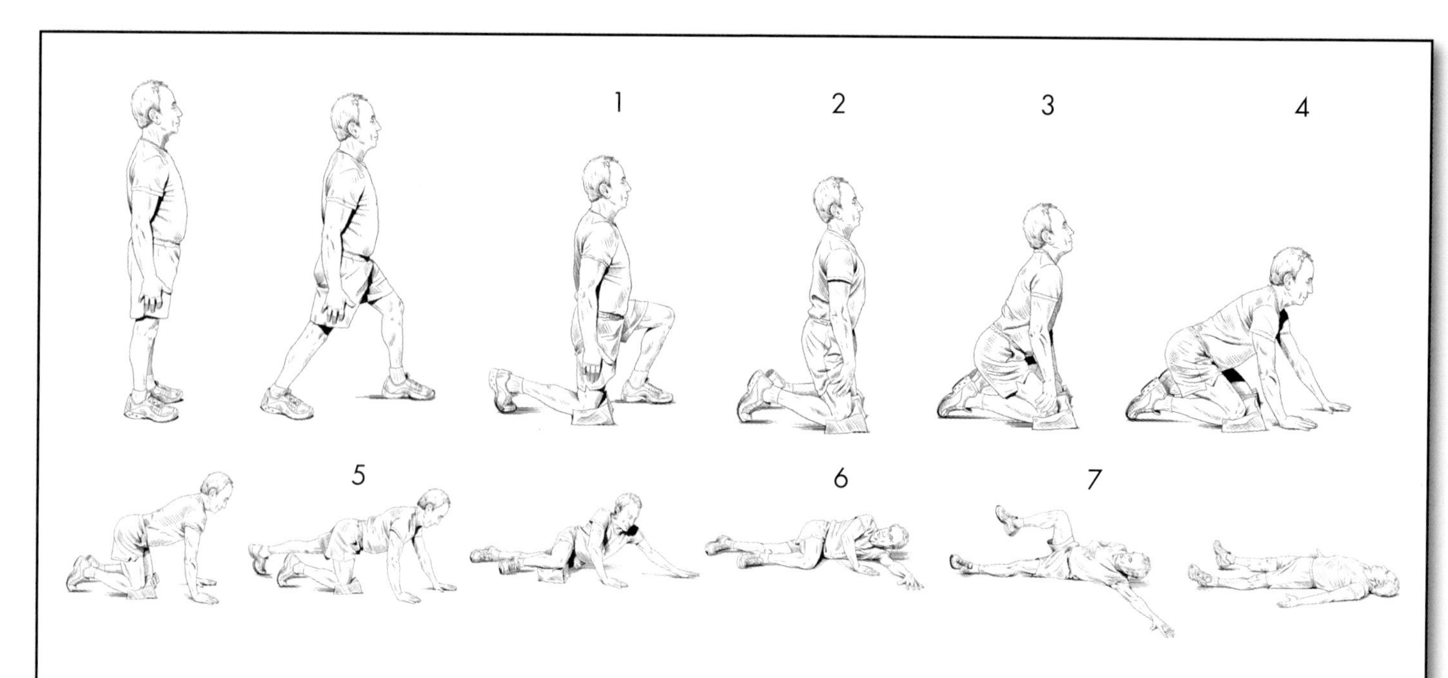

Moving to the floor with the lunge. No spine motion occurs. The spine is stiffened in the "sweet spot" position. Motion occurs at the shoulders and hips.
1. While still maintaining your abdominal brace, take a step forward and drop to one knee.
2. Bring the other knee to the ground all the while controlling spine motion so that no pain is triggered.
3. Slide your hands down the thighs similar to the short-stop squat.
4. Walk your hands forward on the floor until you are supported "on all fours" with your hands and knees.
5. Push one hand forward while dropping the knee of the same side back.
6. Lower the rib cage and hip to the floor maintaining the neutral spine position.
7. Roll over the straight leg onto the back with no spine twist.

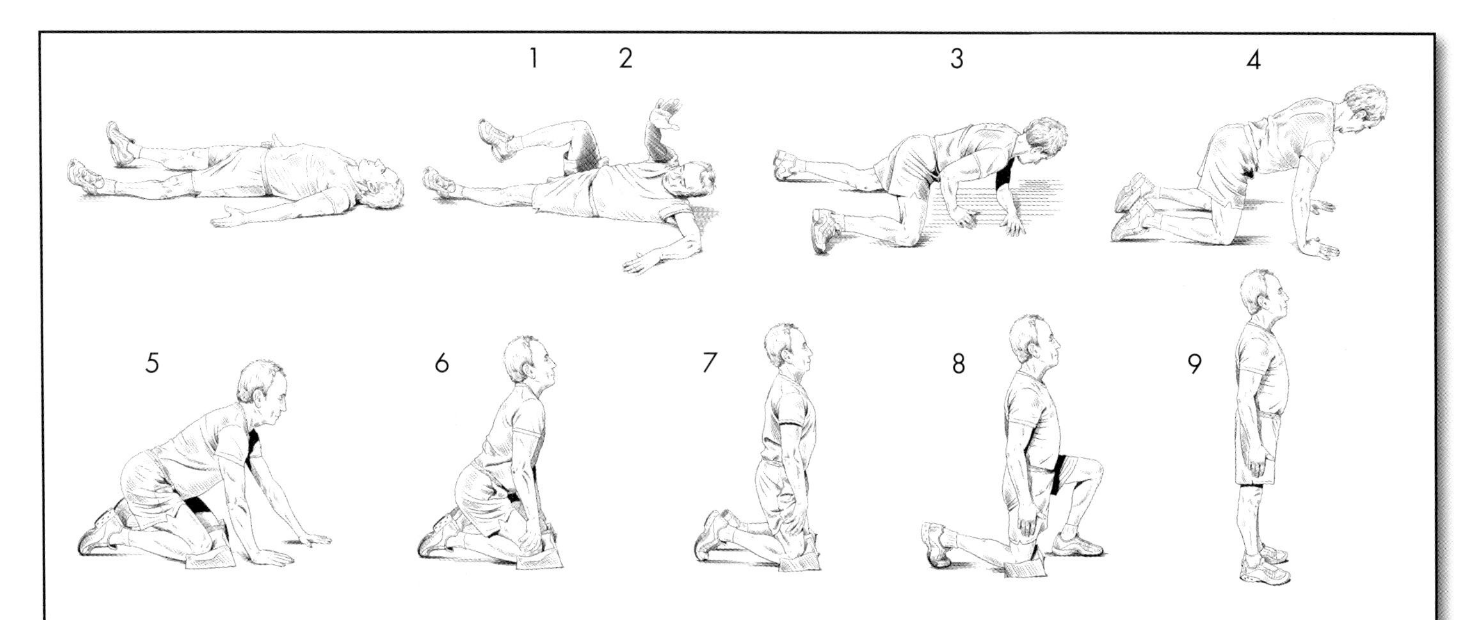

Rising from the floor begins with the "babies crawl" technique of bringing the bent leg over the straight leg. The rib cage is locked in the same position as the pelvis so no spine motion occurs. This should be accomplished pain free.

1. Bend one knee towards you, keeping the other straight.
2. Roll over the straight leg locking the rib cage and pelvis together (to avoid twisting the spine), and plant the knee high on the ground on the other side.
3. Just as you plant the knee, stiffen the shoulder to prop the upper body up on the supporting elbow.
4. Pull other knee through to all fours (hands and knees) with no spine motion.
5. Walk your hands back to your knees.
6. Stiffen your back, pushing down through your arms.
7. Draw your hands up your thighs by pulling your hips forward.
8. Maintaining torso stiffness and control, now place one foot in front of you to prepare the lunge. Be sure to tuck the toes of the rear foot.
9. Initiate leg drive and stand up – all pain free!

Tying your shoes in a way that obeys the principles of spine hygiene requires a modified lunge. Put one foot on a bench, then, most importantly – move the hips towards the elevated foot rather than reaching forward with the back. Now tie the shoe without triggering pain.

3. *The Stop Twist*

This movement tool focuses on preventing twisting motion in your painful back while performing tasks such as opening doors, and rolling over in bed. It also establishes a technique for more pain-free athleticism in the future.

Try the following test to see if you are ready to move on to more advanced training.

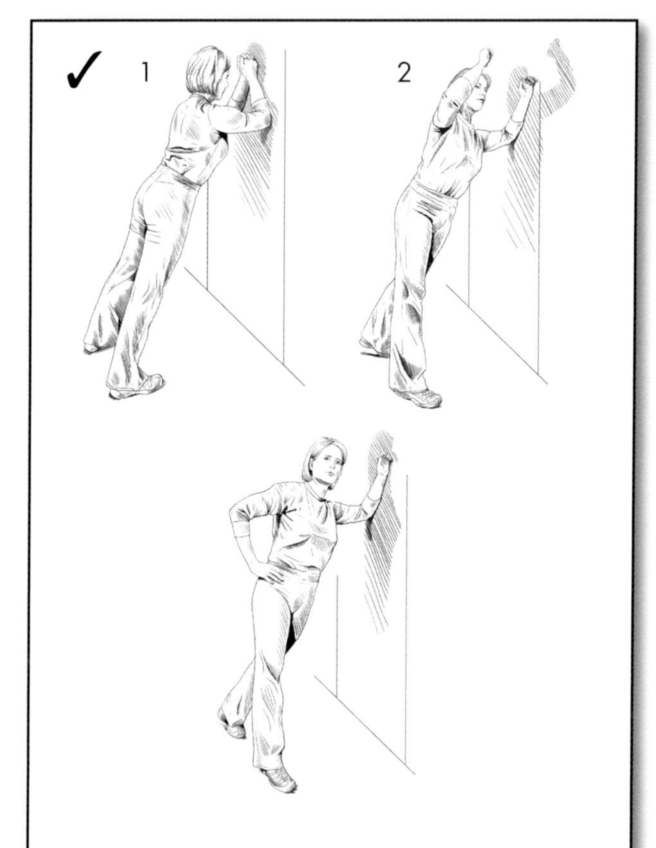

1. Plank on a wall remembering how to find your "sweet spot" posture of the back and hips.
2. Using your toes as a pivot point, roll to a side plank. Watch for the initiation of movement, particularly that motion does not begin with the hips, but rather the hips and ribcage together as a unit. They should continue to move together as you roll, preventing any twisting of the spine.

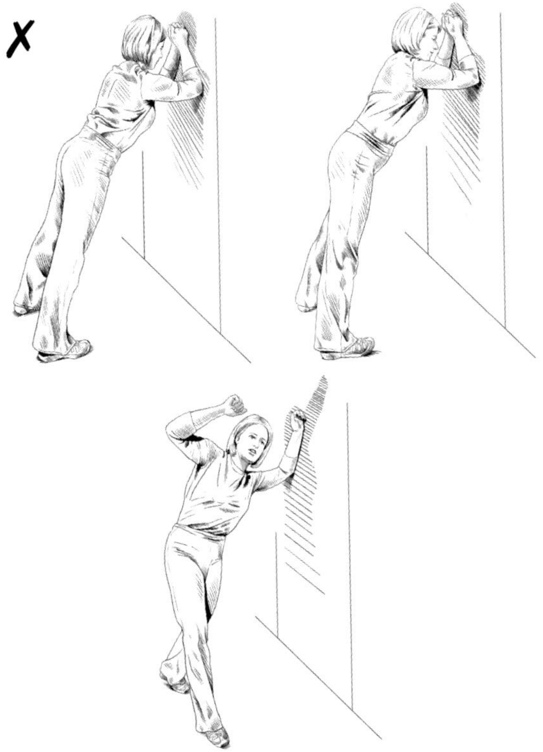

✗

Movement flaws during the "stop twist" include initiating and leading the motion with the pelvis which allows the spine to twist. Correct this by changing the mental thought from "twisting" to stiffening the torso and pulling the locked torso around with the latissimus muscles. Another flaw is losing the straight alignment of the body during the motion – stay tall and aligned.

The Mental Component of Movement Patterns

Being mentally aware and engaged in our movement patterns is fundamental in creating pain-free posture and movement. Your success rests in your ability to move mindfully and to be conscious and aware of your movements. Be aware of your spine posture. Eliminate painful postures.

These exercises will not only help in building that increased mindfulness, but also give you a variety of tools to use while creating a greater pain-free repertoire as you go about your daily routine.

Chapter 8
Spine Hygiene: Expanding Your Pain-Free Abilities

Spine Hygiene

Expanding Your Pain-Free Abilities

Spine hygiene refers to the daily upkeep of your back. It includes your recovery exercise routine as well as changes to your existing daily motions all day long. Success in removing back pain requires removal of the movement flaws that cause tissue stress. The "movement tools" you perfected in the previous chapter should be allowing you to move with less pain. Now we expand your pain-free abilities through the following recommendations. It's time to stop picking at the proverbial scab.

Be forewarned, some of these suggestions go against prevailing wisdom. Yet they are crucial to achieving and maintaining spine health.

Sitting

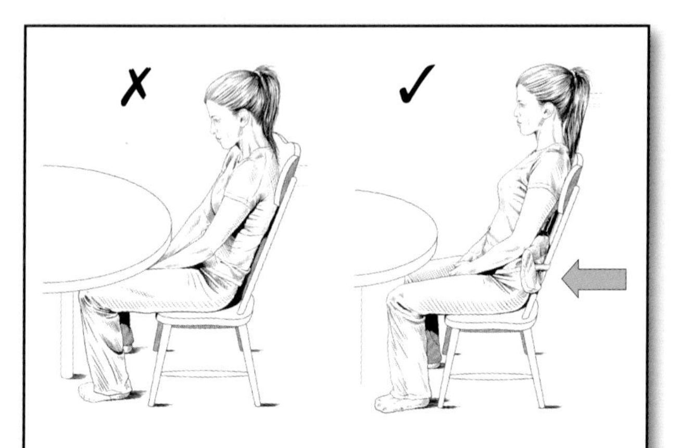

Avoid slouched sitting which stresses the posterior parts of the spine discs. This steals pain-free resilience for the rest of the day. Do sit with the neutral curves of the spine maintained which will build a pain-free back in all other activities. Note the lumbar pad supporting the natural curve of the low back.

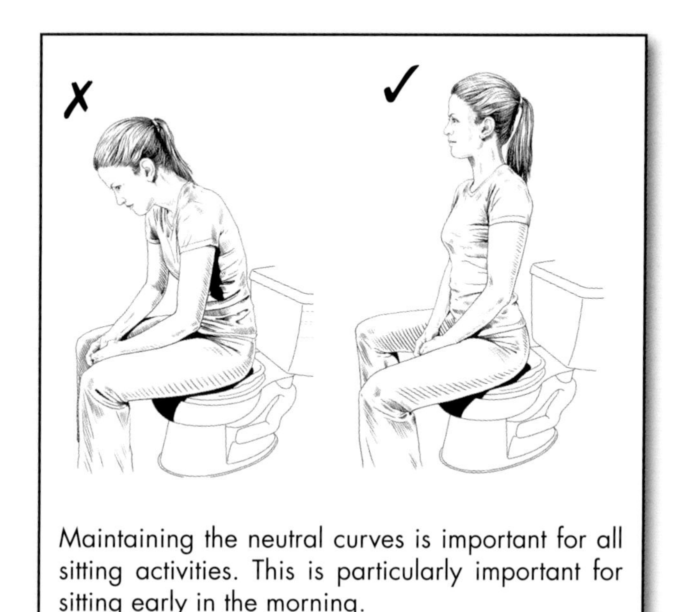

Maintaining the neutral curves is important for all sitting activities. This is particularly important for sitting early in the morning.

Following time spent sitting, many will notice difficulty in standing upright. In fact, it causes much discomfort. Try this drill to regain the stress-free upright standing posture.

We developed this to combat the stresses to the discs that build up during a period of sitting. Use the drill to break up periods of sitting to avoid building up back discomfort. Start with getting up from the chair and repeating every 20 minutes. Then adjust this time interval as you experiment with what works best for you.

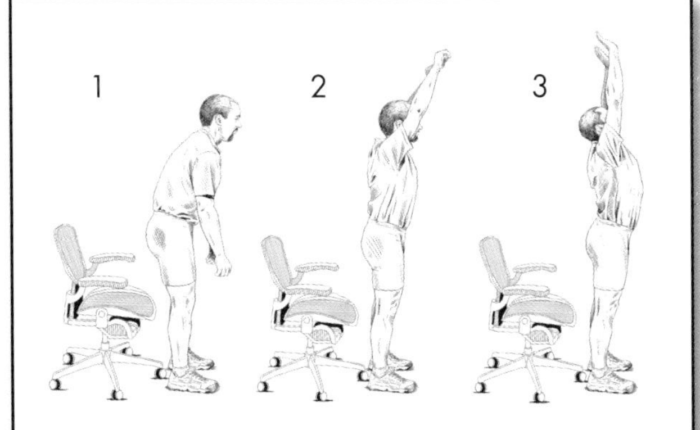

Typically, the back pained person rises from the chair and stands slouched (1). The corrective drill starts with raising the arms overhead, count to 10 (2). Now reach higher and reach farther back for another count of 10 (3). In this position, fully and deeply inhale, working into an upright and stress free standing posture. Drop the arms and relax. Now you have prepared your back to take on the next challenge, be that walking or another sitting session.

Standing

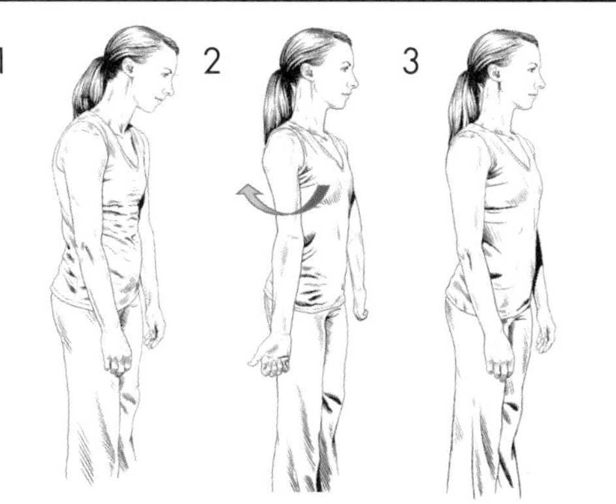

The Drill

Poor standing posture (1) robs pain-free activities by constantly contracting the low back extensor muscles. Try this corrective drill: the thumbs are extended into the hitch-hikers position, then the shoulders are externally rotated lifting the rib cage and posturing the upper body in-line with the hips (2). Now, notice the back muscles relax (3).

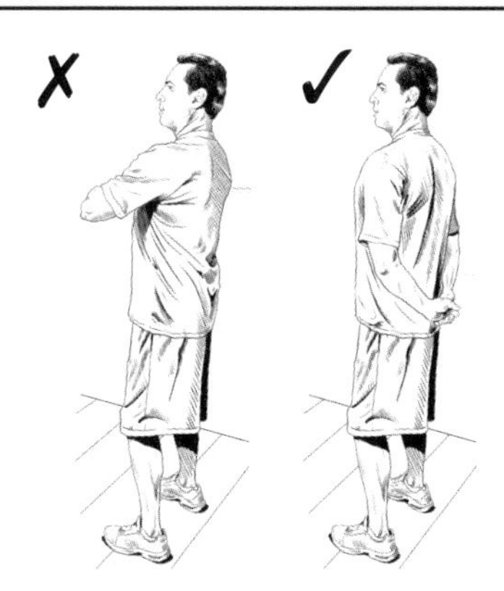

Standing with the arms folded across the chest increases the load on the back muscles and the spine. In contrast, spine hygiene principles include standing with the hands clasped behind the back to reduce muscle activity and the associated cramping.

Walking

Pain causes flexion at the spine and hips resulting in a slouched posture. Slow walking will also cause more pain. Typically the arms are not swung. Walking this way will increase your pain. Change walking into a painfree and enjoyable therapeutic activity. Use some of the drills shown in Chapter 10. Your goal is to create a walking style that takes your pain away.

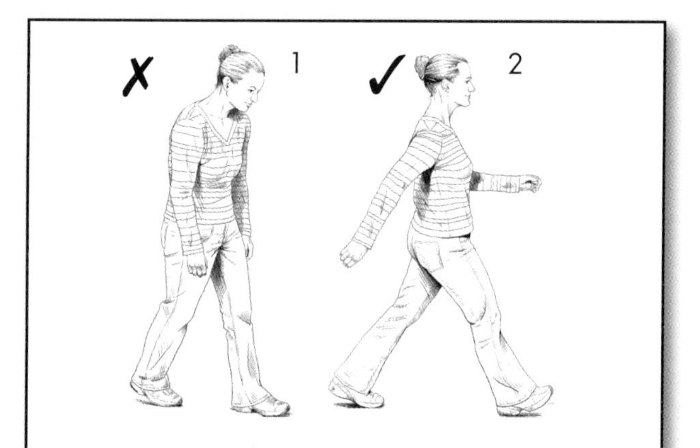

Fix the painful "mall strolling" pattern (1). Instead turn walking into a therapy by correcting your posture to one that is more upright, swing the arms about the shoulders (not the elbows) and take larger and faster steps (2). Use the hints in chapter 10 to create your painfree walking therapy.

Bending

You know the dreaded feeling when faced with the prospect of picking up a sock from the floor. If you're looking for an alternative to the squat in the previous chapter, when bending to pick up relatively light objects, try the "Golfer's lift". This is another pattern in which motion comes from the hips, not the back. Avoiding spine flexion means avoiding many potential pain triggers.

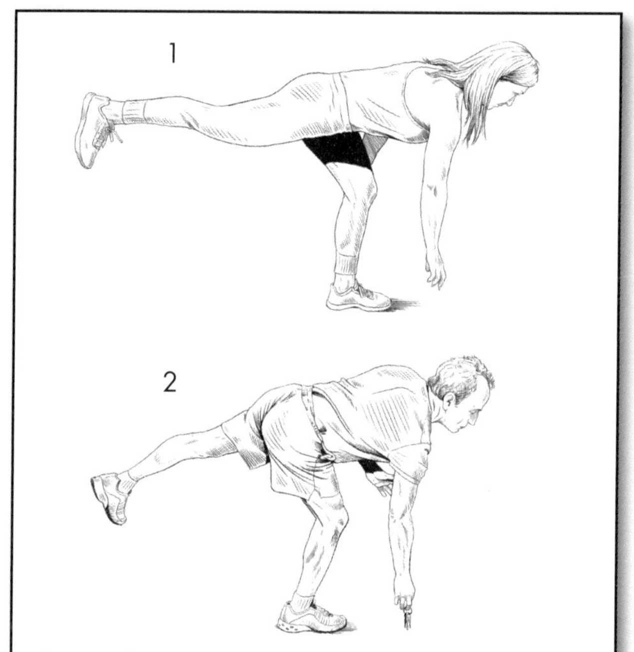

The Golfers Lift preserves the "sweet spot" and pain-free spine posture while picking up light objects from the floor. Begin by standing in your neutral, pain-free posture. Now, bend at the stance hip, moving your torso forward while keeping the back flat, you will be able to reach the floor! For proper balance, as your torso moves forward, extend one of your legs straight out behind you to act as a counter-weight. You may hold a chair or other sturdy object with the non-reaching hand. Practice this move for balance and no pain. Some find more comfort reaching with the arm opposite to the support leg (1), yet others prefer the same side arm (2).

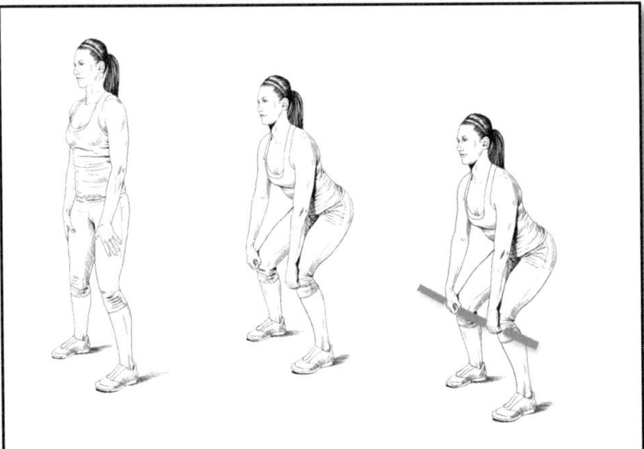

Recall the short-stop squat or hip-hinge style. Incorporate the "anti-shrug" pattern to stiffen the back in a pain-free posture. This is adapted to all squats and bends including lifting.

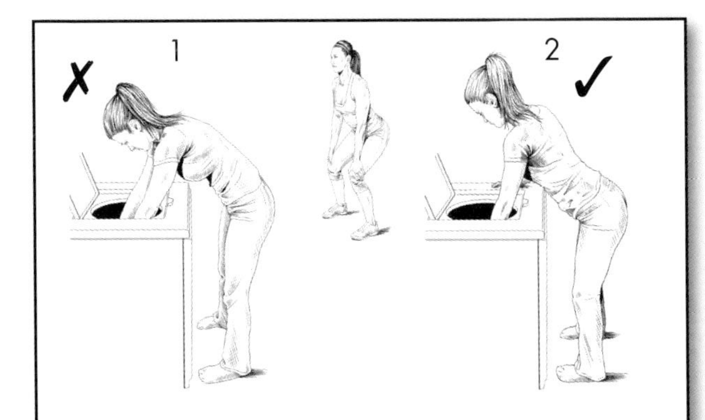

All daily activities are opportunities to spare the spine or make it sensitive to pain – the choice is yours. Here the hand (2) is supporting the back while one hand gathers the laundry with a neutral spine. Complete the task to upright standing with the anti-shrug, hip-hinge technique.

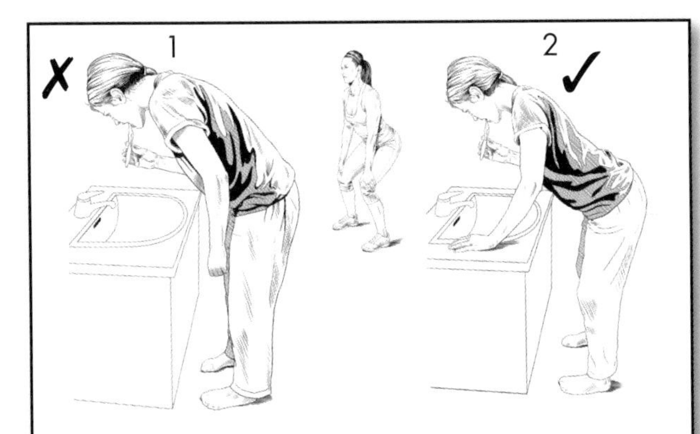

Brushing the teeth without hip-hinging stresses the discs making them painful (1). Begin with the hip-hinge, sliding your hands down the thighs. Then place one hand on the counter-top, and brush your teeth with the other (2). When finished, place one hand on one knee, then the other hand to knee and perform the stiffening "anti-shrug". Now "pull the hips through". You are building pain-free resilience.

Pushing and Pulling

Next time you are in an office space or a commercial building with a heavy door, examine how you push against it. If there's one in the building in which you are currently reading, get up and try it before proceeding to read. Go ahead, do it.

Now review your mental checklist from before the push. Did you fine-tune the stiffening of your abdominal muscles to just the right amount? While maintaining an upright torso, did you then reach and pull with your shoulder muscles as opposed to twisting through your torso? Did you step around the door only releasing the brace after letting go of the door?

When pushing or pulling, another key principle is to direct the force from the hand right though the navel. In other words, the pathway of pushing or pulling should draw a line either directly towards or directly away from the center of your core.

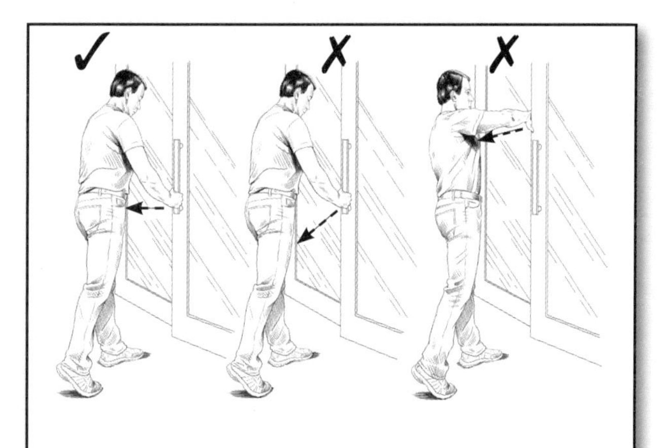

Pull the door with force directed through the spine (the navel provides a good target). Poor technique creates forces not through the spine, causing pain.

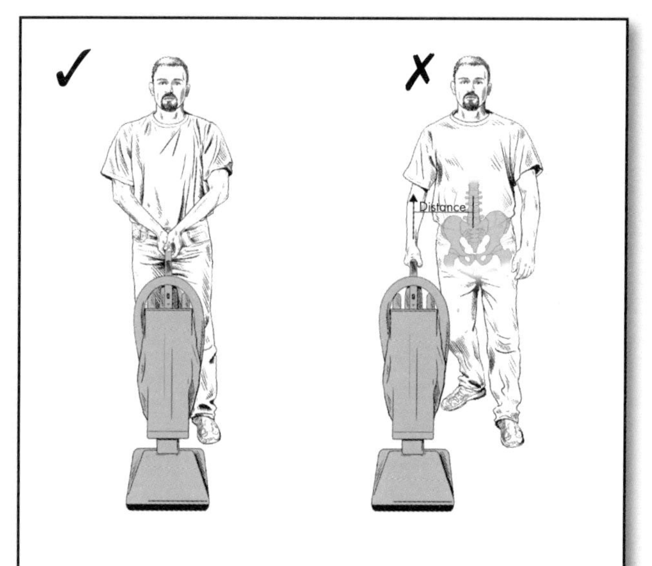

Traditional one-arm vacuuming causes pain in many people. Observe the "distance" of the pushing force, it does not pass through the spine causing crushing muscle activity. Instead "waltz" with the vacuum directing force through the spine – pain-free!

More Spine hygiene: Do Not Allow Pain into Your Back

Now that we've added some more healthy movement adaptations to our list of spine-sparing techniques, here is a checklist of principles to formalize what you have learned thus far. The keys to practicing good spine hygiene include:

- ***Employ a variety of postures:*** You are now aware of the postures that cause your pain. When in one of these postures, adjust it to your optimal position before the pain begins. For example, if sitting is tolerable for 10 minutes before pain can be expected, then change to a standing posture at eight minutes. Or, consider an alternate posture such as kneeling for a short period of time. Even for people who don't usually experience back pain, prolonged periods in one position may cause them grief. The key is to mix it up as much as you can throughout the day, while sparing your spine of course.

- ***Prepare for more load by adjusting your spine posture:*** As an example, next time your are expecting a sneeze, prepare with a resilient posture. Likewise when lifting, preserve the natural curve in your back by avoiding spine rotation and bending at the hips. This concept implies that you should not repeatedly pick up objects from the floor, if you are trying to preserve your spine. If you find that you must pick up a light object repeatedly from the floor consider the golfers lift shown previously. Recall tying your shoe, a squat pattern will not work, nor will a sitting posture allow you to obey the pain-free principles.

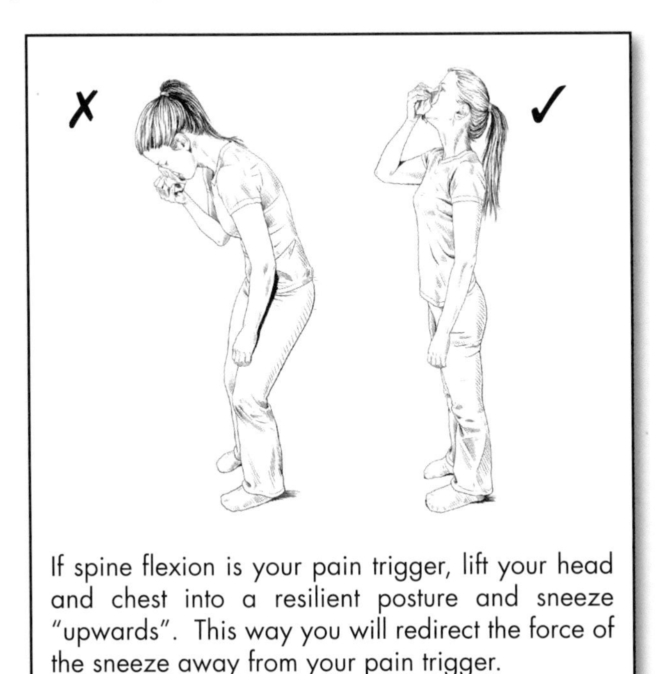

If spine flexion is your pain trigger, lift your head and chest into a resilient posture and sneeze "upwards". This way you will redirect the force of the sneeze away from your pain trigger.

- ***Choose postures to minimize loads on your body:*** Recall how holding an object away from your body places more load on your back muscles and thus more load on your spine. Therefore when carrying, lifting or moving objects, hold them as close to your body as possible. (keep the hand loads close).
- ***Strategically alter a task to minimize the actual weight of the load being handled:*** In some tasks it is possible to just lift one half of the object at a time (for example, positioning boxes up on one corner or lifting only one end of an object such as a log). Don't overburden yourself when there is the option to lift smarter.

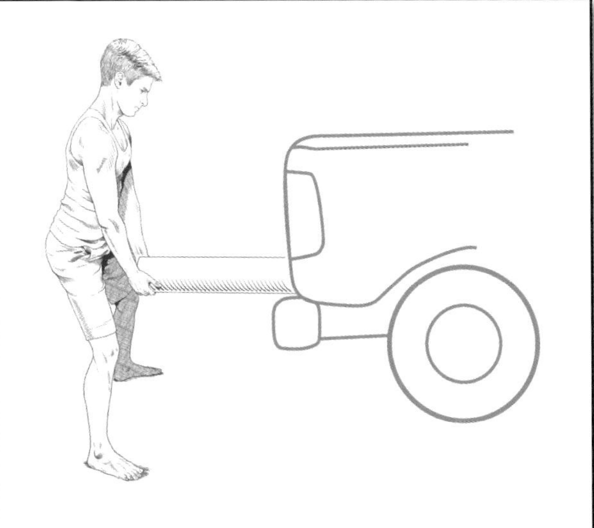

When lifting a large object, avoid picking up the entire weight in its middle. Here just one end of a log is picked up and placed in the truck bed. Then the other end is lifted in. The log was lifted by only ever taking half its weight.

- ***Avoid immediate strenuous exertions after a prolonged activity such as sitting or stooping:*** Your spinal discs need a minute or two to "equilibrate" stress. For example, if you have been gardening or sitting for a while, don't stand up and lift immediately. Do stand and walk for a few minutes in order to rebalance the spinal discs and to minimize stress and pain. Recall the restoring drill following sitting earlier in this chapter.
- ***Avoid lifting or spine bending shortly after rising from bed:*** The risk of injury is higher at this time of day because the discs are swollen. Example: Get dressed by bending at the hips: Avoid exercises such as sit-ups or the infamous "pulling the knees to the chest stretch" early in the morning. This is something often mistakenly recommended for morning stiffness.
- ***Stiffen your core appropriately:*** This technique often eliminates the micro-movements in your spine that trigger pain. Remember to stiffen the abdominal wall like a dimmer switch. The important element is to match the effort of stiffening to the task. More contraction is required for heavier tasks. Develop the ability to deliver just enough to control the pain trigger for "light" tasks.

- ***Avoid twisting of the spine when exerting force:*** Example: Avoid exercises that cause spine loading (and muscle activity) while twisting such as the bodybuilder's "Russian twist" exercise. Choose work techniques that control spinal motion when twisting.

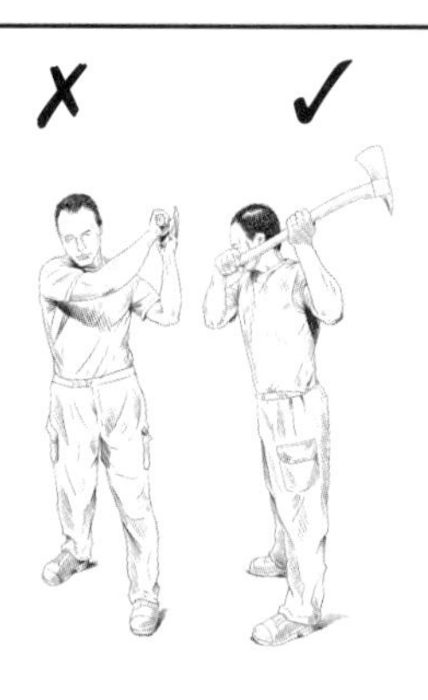

Poor technique allows spine twist while generating twisting torque (where the muscles are trying to forcefully untwist the spine). This causes high spine stress. Good technique does not allow spine twist.

The spine is locked and motion occurs in the shoulders and hips.

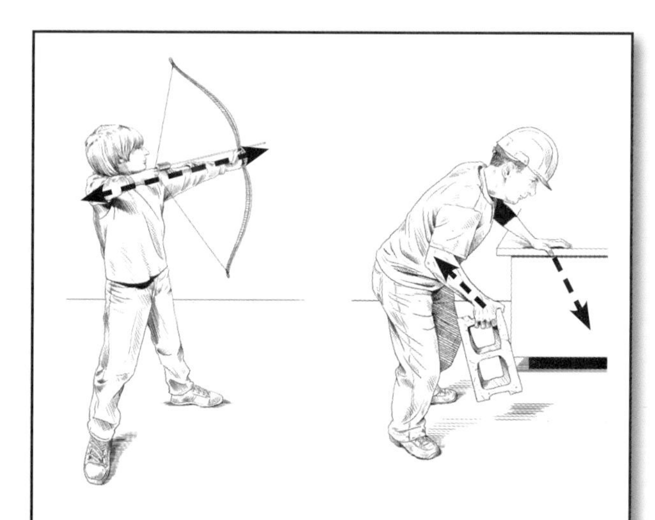

Archers bow principle: A bow and arrow requires a push with one arm and a pull with the other. The spine remains neutral. Adapting the technique to lift objects follows the principles of spine hygiene.

- ***Use momentum when exerting force to reduce the spine load:*** This is in contrast to the often heard recommendation "always lift slowly and smoothly" – this is an ill-founded recommendation for many skilled workers. It is safer to generate momentum in the torso first and transfer it to an object being moved as long as the spine is stiffened in a neutral posture.

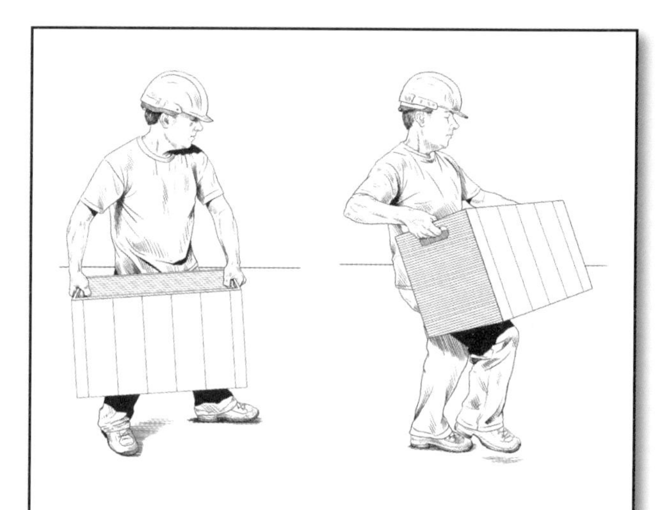

Saddle toss principle: Imagine lifting a saddle onto a horses' back slowly and smoothly – this would cause pain! Replace that ill-founded recommendation with good cowboy skill. Here the saddle is placed against the knee and the leg creates momentum to "throw" the saddle up, sparing the back. Adapt this technique to different objects.

- ***Avoid prolonged sitting:*** This goes back to the idea of varying your postures but it is worth repeating. Whether in the car, at the office, or on the couch, it is important to take standing and walking breaks to help alleviate your back strain. And, use a lumbar support if you have flexion intolerance.
- ***Consider the best rest break strategies:*** One size does not fit all meaning that breaks have to be customized for different jobs and tasks. The break should be the mechanical opposite of the task demands. Example: If dynamic work is performed, sit for a break. If the task requires sitting then the rest break should be walking. If your job requires sitting you must walk on your breaks and at lunch.

- ***Consider the right accessories to foster joint conserving postures:*** Example, if kneeling reduces the need to stoop through your back, then use knee pads. If dirty, or sharp edged and heavy objects are to be lifted and carried, use a leather apron to hold the load close to your body.
- ***Plan movements before executing them:*** Plot your movements to spare joints, reduce distances travelled, and back up distal joint movement with stiffness at the proximal joints. These carefully executed patterns will soon become second nature and you will be able to spare your back without even thinking about it.
- ***Maintain an appropriate level of general fitness:*** This means that all components of fitness are in balance with one another (flexibility/stiffness, strength, endurance, power, balance, stability/mobility, and movement skill) to steer forces through the body linkages in a joint sparing way.

To Summarize

At this point, you have years of movement habits to break. Unconscious movement patterns need to be unlearned and replaced. Through the continued use of good spine hygiene, the overheated central nervous system will have time to cool. You have begun the pain desensitization process that will ensure a pain-free future.

Be mindful to adhere to the spine sparing movement principles presented here until they become your new habits. If your focus or concentration lapses, you can bet that pain will return to remind you of your inattention. Rest assured that over time pain-free alternative movement patterns will come naturally.

Chapter 9

Building a Resilient Back: The Non-Negotiable "Big 3" Exercises

Building a Resilient Back

The Non-Negotiable "Big 3" Exercises

Essential Exercises for Everyone

At this point in your reading you should have a comprehensive understanding of which triggers to avoid and how to modify your daily motions as you work to "wind down" your pain.

We will now begin exercises that will enhance your back fitness and set the stage to broaden your range of pain-free activities.

By exercises, I don't mean hour-long workouts at the gym; far from it! What I recommend as a first step to every back sufferer looking to build their fitness and pain-free function is to practice what I call the "Big 3." These are:

1. The modified curl-up
2. The side bridge
3. The birddog/quadruped

Our research showed these exercises were superior for their ability to spare the back while building muscular fitness and maintaining stability and control. They are able to prevent painful joint micro-movements for several hours. They also build endurance, an essential component in adding activities back into your lifestyle that previously caused pain.

The "Big 3" have a few common features. While performing the following "routine", it is essential that you find your appropriate starting level then progress from there. Training times begin with 10 second position holds. This short holding time reduces the risk of triggering muscle cramp pain. Use my "descending pyramid" model to guide your repetitions and sets. Work to build up endurance with repeated, short, exercise bouts: this means avoiding engaging in infrequent and/or extended sessions of long duration. For example, if you can't exercise for 10 minutes without pain then try three sessions over the day lasting six minutes each. This accomplishes a total of 18 minutes of pain-free training!

Remember to avoid being that extreme Type A or Type B patient. Instead, strive to be a Type C exerciser: a Competent Exerciser. Nothing fancy: just follow the instructions and you will make progress. As you enhance your pain-free training capacity, you can gradually shift to longer, fewer sessions each day. Your progression to more difficult versions of these three exercises is dependent upon your ability to master the tecnhique of the basic exercises *first*.

Once you've mastered the "Big 3", you can progress to more difficult versions of these three exercises. As I'm sure you've discovered by now, each chapter sets a base knowledge in order to continue to the next. The "Big 3" are no exception. Your success in performing the exercises in the following chapters depends upon your ability to perform these basic three.

FIVE IMPORTANT TIPS

1. **You must practice these exercises daily.**
2. **Avoid performing these immediately after rising from bed. The optimal time would be mid-morning to dinnertime.** Most people are not fresh enough to reap the benefits when performing these exercises right before bedtime either.
3. **Choosing the dose of exercise within a single session is supremely important.** The most tender backs will only tolerate very short sessions of exercise and thus will benefit most from several, very brief, sessions throughout the day. If the exercises are too much in one session, split the number of exercises into two halves, one session in the morning and one in the afternoon. There will be some people who begin with three or even four very short sessions daily. As they progress, the sessions slowly are reduced to one per day with an appropriate increase in dosage.
4. **Bracing the abdominal muscles, rather than hollowing or sucking them in, during exercise invokes all of the advantages of achieving a stable core.** To brace, tighten the entire core, "tuning" the effort to reduce pain.
5. **Try and maintain your spine in the pain-free posture.** Create motion about the shoulders and hips, not the spine.

The Big 3

1. The Curl-up

This curl-up is light years away from a standard abdominal crunch exercise. And, to be clear, sit-ups should simply have no place in the exercise plan of a back patient.

The setup: During the curl-up there should be no movement through the lumbar spine. When lying down on the floor face-up, slide your hands under your low back to support the lumbar spine. This position will prevent the lower spine from flattening against the floor and minimize the stress on your back. Keeping one leg extended, bring the other up into a bent position, with the foot planted in line with the knee of the extended leg.

Curl-up technique: Begin by stiffening the abdominal muscles just enough to prevent motion but not to cause any pain. Elevate your elbows off the floor so that they "float" at your sides, your hands still under your lumbar region. Maintain a neutral spine (including the neck) and slightly lift only the head and shoulders off the floor. It is important to keep the neck (cervical spine) and lower torso (lumbar spine) as immobile as possible. When performing the exercise simply raise the head and shoulders off the ground, count to 10 then lower your back to the starting position. It may help to consider your head and shoulders resting on a bathroom scale – now make the scale show zero weight. Thus, compared to a crunch, the curl-up involves minimal movement. To an outsider it may not look like you're doing much of anything, but with the proper technique applied, you should feel like you're working. It is important to practice deep breathing during the actual exercise.

Prescription: Experiment with five repetitions (of about 8-10 seconds long each), then rest for about 30 seconds. Next try three repetitions, then rest, then one repetition – you are finished. See how you feel the following day. If you are doing well, you may add one repetition to each set – in this case increasing them to six reps, four reps and two reps respectively. (Notice the descending reps with each set – this is the Russian descending pyramid). If you have no leg pain, alternate the bent leg with each set. If you experience leg or buttock pain then bend the knee on the side that proves painful.

THE RUSSIAN DESCENDING PYRAMID FOR SETS AND REPS PROGRAM DESIGN

This very clever system guides the number of sets and reps to build some endurance without getting fatigued, and it helps prevent muscular cramps by restoring the oxygen and acid balance every 8-10 seconds. I learned it from Russian masters and honour them with the name. Typically there are 3 sets. The holds are 8-10 seconds long. The first set may be 6 holds with a brief rest (rest a few seconds) between each hold. Now rest perhaps 20-30 seconds. For the second set the number of reps is less – usual 2 less, so the reps in this example will be 4. Rest again for 20 seconds. For the third set subtract 2 more reps – in this example the reps will be 2. Now move on to the next exercise and repeat the descending pyramid.

When more challenge is desired, add 1 rep to each set – do not add to the holding time. Use this when you have pain. As you get out of pain you may go to longer holds and alternate rep/set designs.

Here is an example:

1 rep = 10 second hold

Set 1: 6 reps, rest 20 seconds

Set 2: 4 reps, rest 20 seconds

Set 3: 2 reps, finished

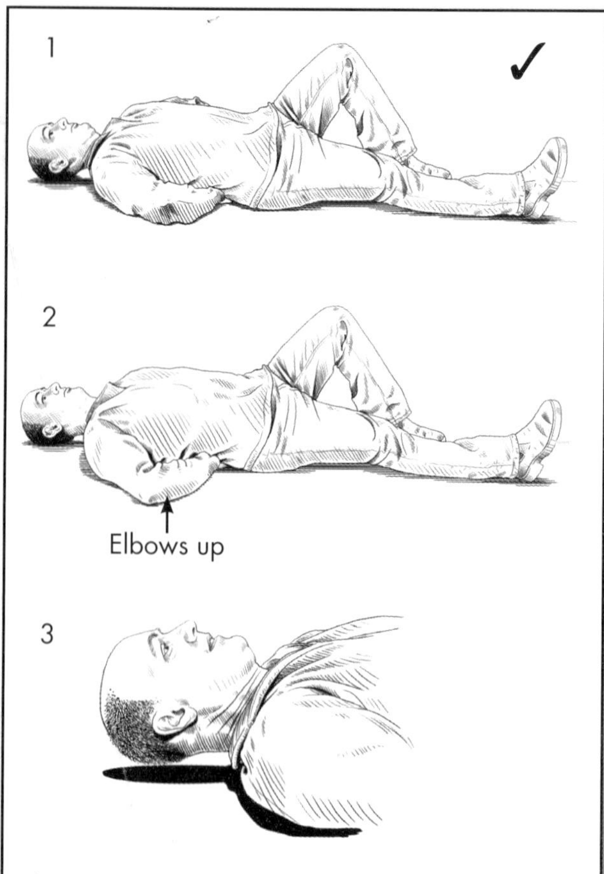

The curl-up. Set-up requires the hands (palms down) under the lumbar region (1). The elbows are raised slightly to not touch the floor (2). The abdominal muscles are braced – the level of the brace is "tuned" by the individual to create the appropriate resistance challenge. The head/neck/shoulders are raised slightly – movement is minimal (3).

REMEDIAL NECK EXERCISES

Some individuals will experience neck discomfort during the curl-up. The likelihood of this is greater in habitual gum chewers, people with long necks and those who have had excessive neck manipulations. Resist the urge to clasp the hands behind the head. Instead, build neck stability and the ability to perform pain-free neck support using this technique:

After you have built up your neck stamina over time, return to the curl-up and try the following technique: Encourage the neck flexors to engage by lightly touching the teeth together. Then push the tongue to the roof of the mouth. Notice the neck flexors engaging under the chin. This corrective technique should reduce your neck discomfort. Side note: did you know that chewing gum might be inhibiting your neck flexors?

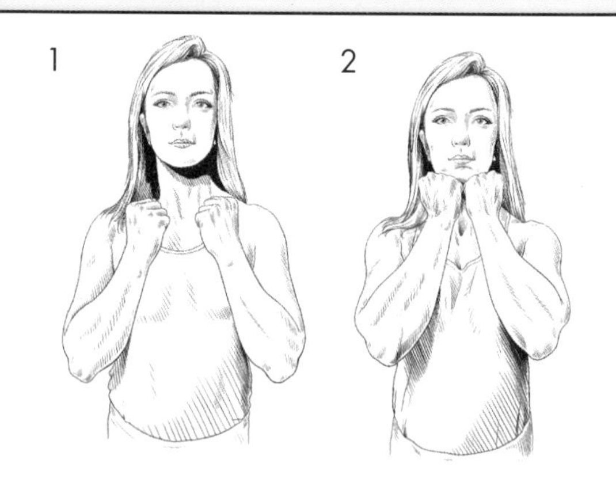

Neck pre-habilitation begins while standing, posturing the head in a neutral pose looking straight ahead, place the fists under the chin. (1) Touch the teeth lightly together and place the tongue to the roof of the mouth behind the teeth. Now push the tongue up to the roof and stiffen the front of the neck. This activates the flexors of the neck and will make the curl-up more comfortable. Gently push the fists upwards while resisting with the neck muscles. No motion occurs (2).
Do this with enough effort to engage the muscles but not to create discomfort or pain. Build the capacity to support your neck in a pain-free manner as you slowly increase the effort.

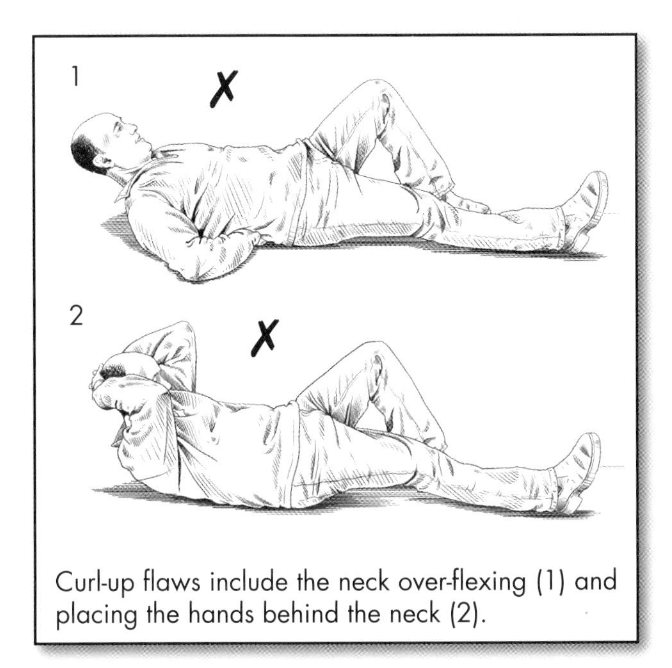

Curl-up flaws include the neck over-flexing (1) and placing the hands behind the neck (2).

2. The Side Bridge or Side Plank

The side bridge family of exercises is unique in that they challenge the critical spine stabilizing muscles. It is one of the few exercises that works to integrate the quadratus lumborum muscle together with the abdominal wall. It does so in a very spine conserving way by keeping one side of the lateral spine musculature relatively "quiet", while the other is active. It also integrates the important latissimus dorsi muscle.

The set-up: The side bridge (or side plank) can be performed from the knees if you have limited strength or an inability to engage the abdominal wall without pain. Begin by lying on your right side supported by the right elbow, hip and outer leg.

Side bridge technique: To prepare to perform a left side bridge place your left elbow on the floor while having your knees bent about ninety degrees. From this position hip-hinge forward similar to a squat. Your right hand (top hand) can rest on the top of your right hip/thigh. Progressions include performing the side bridge so that the feet and elbow are the only contact points, changing your arm position so that your hand is resting on your hips and finally, the rolling side bridge.

Prescription: Hold the bridge for 10 seconds while maintaining normal breathing. Try three or four holds on one side, then repeat on the other side. Add reps until you are close to using up your pain-free capacity, but do not exceed six to start. Rest. Then repeat but perform two fewer reps than before. Rest. Try a third set but reduce the number of reps by another two. Finish. Notice the "descending pyramid" guide to sets and reps. As you continue to improve over time, progress through the forms of side bridge that increase the challenge. When you are performing the full side bridge that involves supporting with the feet and elbow, hold one side 10 seconds, roll to the forward plank on the elbows with no spine twist, hold for three seconds, then roll to the other side. That is one repetition. Try to build to six reps. Then complete the descending pyramid with another four reps, rest, two reps, and finish.

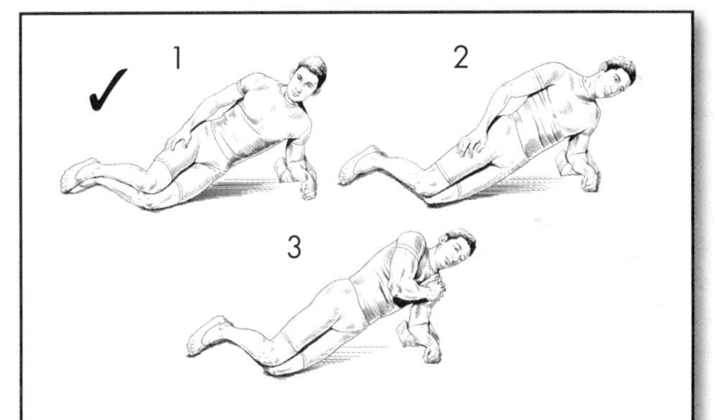

Beginners side bridge. On the floor, the knees and hips are slightly flexed (1). Instead of laterally lifting the pelvis off the floor, the hips are extended in a squat pattern (hip hinge and push the hips forward). The body from the knees up is aligned (2). Those who experience shoulder discomfort will enjoy the technique of placing the "big hand" (fingers spread apart) over the shoulder muscles of the opposite side and pulling the elbow down across the chest (3).

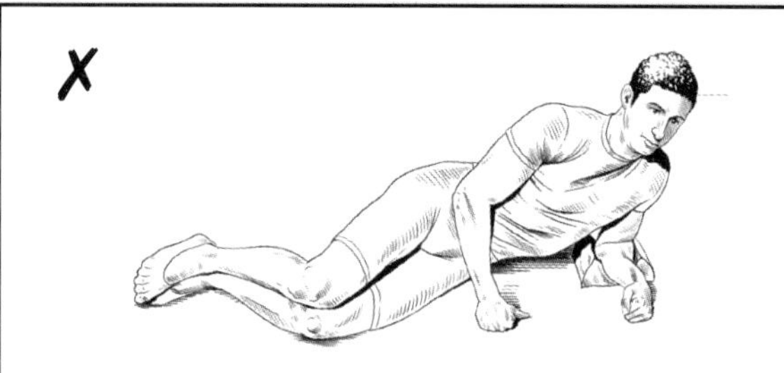

Resist the sloppy resting position where the spine is bent. Instead straighten and align the pelvis and hips while resting to remain pain-free.

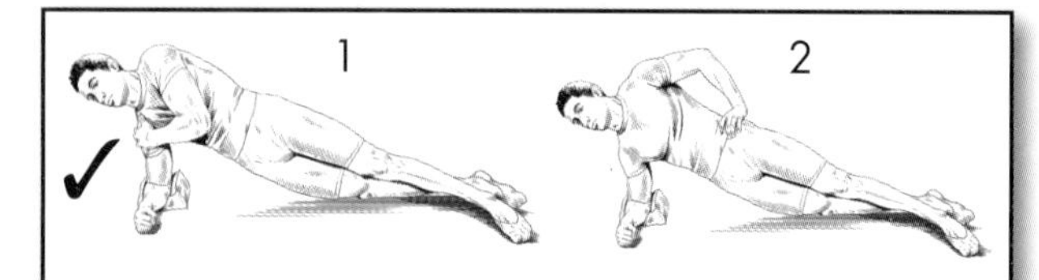

Progress the side bridge by supporting the body using the elbow and feet as contact points with the floor. Notice that the top foot is placed in front of the bottom foot. First, the hand caps the deltoid muscle of the shoulder and the elbow is pulled down across the chest. This relieves the shoulder of discomfort (1). Further, more mass can be added to the "bridge" by placing the hand on the waist increasing the challenge (2).

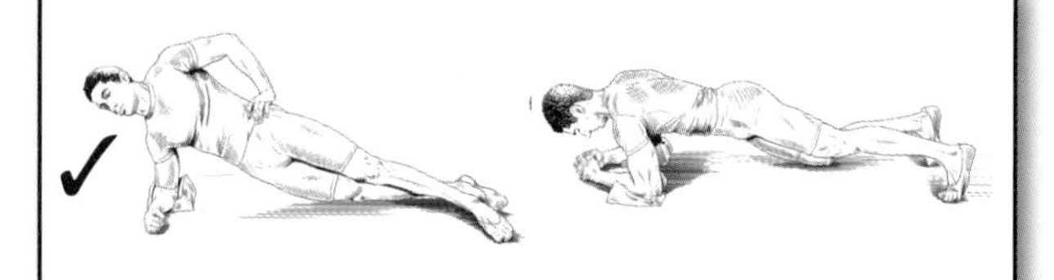

The side bridge may be progressed to incorporate a "roll". Here the torso is stiffened and the motion takes place only about the shoulders and hips. Once in the front plank, the roll is continued to the other side for a 10 second hold.

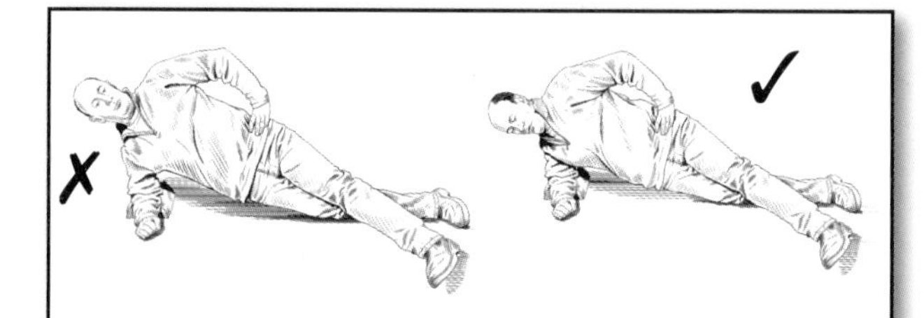

Movement flaws during the roll include initiating the movement with the pelvis causing a twist in the spine. Go back to the "torsional buttress" and eliminate this flaw – lock and stiffen the ribcage to the pelvis and concentrate on creating the motion with the latissimus dorsi muscle.

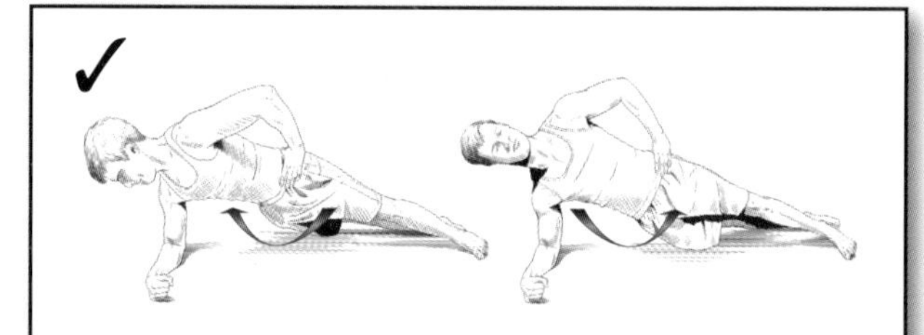

Once the flawless side plank is mastered, different neuromuscular compartments of the abdominal wall can be activated and challenged in this advanced technique by subtly rolling the navel towards the floor then reversing to roll up towards the ceiling while facing sideways. Ensure the motion occurs about the shoulder and not with spine twist. The torso remains a block.

REMEDIAL EXERCISES

If the side bridge on the floor is too challenging or painful at first, pull back to this version:

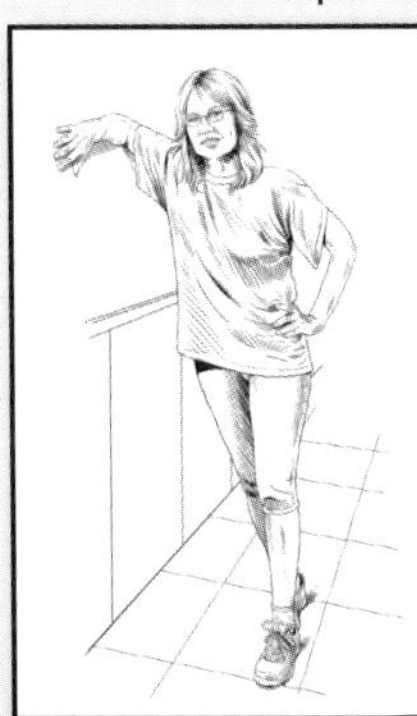

The wall plank: Lean against a wall. Place the outside foot in front and move the spine and hips in such a way as to find a pain-free posture. Build the 10-second holds with sets and reps similar to the floor side bridge.

The side bridge for those with compromised shoulders

Some of you will be unable to support your weight due to shoulder injury and pain. I have had patients who are NFL linebackers who fit into this group, so not bearing weight with the shoulders is not about weakness, but the existence of pain. Though the following exercise is not as beneficial as the side bridge, it is worth trying for those in need of a more basic variation. Lie on your side. Stiffen your abdominals and slightly raise both legs just off the floor.

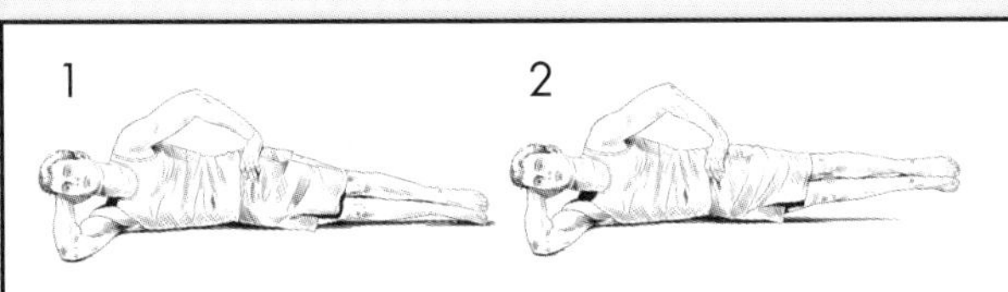

While lying on your side, find the spine's natural curves (1). Appropriately brace your abdominal muscles. (2) Slightly lift your legs while ensuring minimal spine bending. The image of just barely making the scale under the legs weigh zero works well to perfect the technique.

3. The Bird-Dog

This exercise not only targets the back but also the hip extensors. It also teaches the discipline of using proper hip and shoulder motion while maintaining a stable spine.

Our research has shown that employing the bird-dog exercise spares the spine from high compressive loads and ensures stable patterns of muscle activity. It challenges both lumbar and thoracic portions of multiple major back muscles (the longissimus, iliocostalis, and multifidus). This exercise is also a major contributor in desensitizing back pain!

The set-up: While on all fours, position the spine into its most resilient position, moving with subtle flexion/extension movement. In this way the lumbar spine is placed into a pain-free "sweet spot." The thoracic spine is curved slightly upward. The hips are flexed with the knees contacting the floor directly under the hips. The hands are under the shoulders. Appropriately stiffen the abdominals to control the torso and to ensure that motion will be focused solely around the hips and shoulders.

Bird-dog technique: Kneel down on all fours and then raise the opposite arm and leg simultaneously. Do not raise the arm higher than the shoulder nor the leg past the height of the hips. The objective is to be able to hold the limbs parallel to the floor for about six to eight seconds. The bird-dog is improved by "sweeping" the upraised hand and knee along the floor in between "holds." This is called "sweep the floor" and should not involve bearing any weight on either the hand or the foot in motion. Remember that the spine is locked while only the shoulder and hip joints are moving.

Muscle contraction through the upper back can be enhanced during this exercise by clenching the upraised fist. To further target the low back, gluteal and hamstring muscles, try pushing the heel away while keeping the foot flexed (ie. the opposite of pointing your toes). This will also reduce the tendency for "hip hiking," a motion that twists the spine.

A more basic version of the bird-dog posture can be used by those with extremely tender backs. For this modified bird-dog posture we raise just one leg, no arm. Emphasize abdominal bracing and a neutral spine regardless of the variation you choose.

When you've mastered the basic "hold and sweep" pattern of repetitions, it's time to progress to "drawing squares". While in the "hold" position, laterally draw the fist away from the midline and concentrate on arm extension. The foot follows the same pattern as the hand. Specifically, draw the hand/foot out and away, down, across to the midline, and up to the start position. The square should be no larger than a foot (30 cm) in size. The activity of the upper extensors, rhomboids, latissimus dorsi and lower trapezius will be greatly enhanced by this simple fist clinching movement.

Prescription: Create a set/rep program based on a descending pyramid. For example try four, 10-second holds on the right side, then repeat on the left. Rest about 30 seconds, now perform three reps on each side, and rest, then repeat two reps on each side. Then finish. When more challenge is needed, add one rep to each set, do not increase the 10-second holding time. Eventually you may work to longer holding times once your back pain has diminished.

The bird-dog prescription usually follows a similar set/rep/rest configuration as the side bridge.

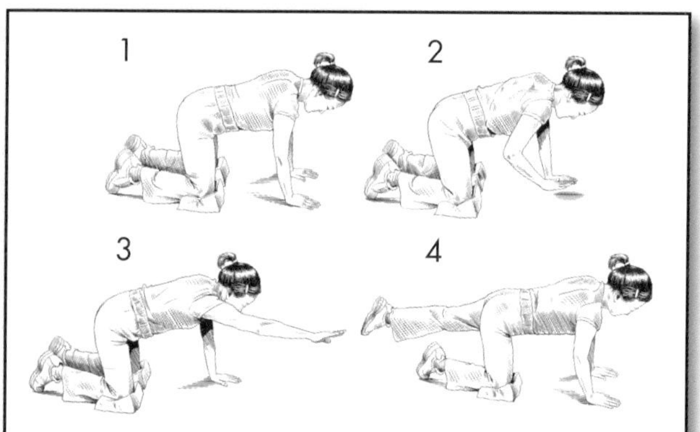

For the most pained people, bird-dog progressions begin on the hands and knees. Effort is directed towards finding the "sweet spot" spine position, the shoulders over the hands (1), the hips over the knees. As with all exercises, these must be performed pain-free. Some will need to begin by simply raising a hand by bending one elbow (2). Hold for 10 seconds. Then progress to extending the arm (3), and then one leg at a time (4). Raise it to the point of challenge but no pain.

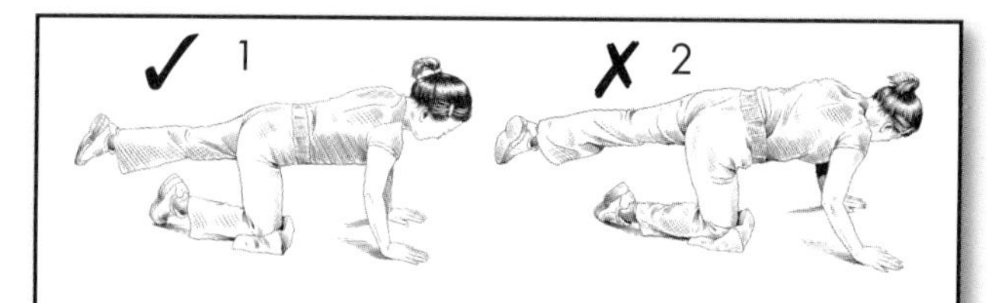

Be aware of movement flaws such as allowing the spine to twist (2) which will eventually cause pain and thwart progress to the more challenging levels.

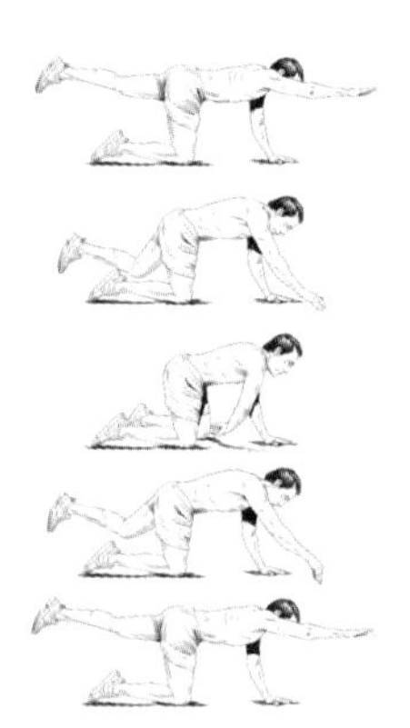

The progression continues with the "sweep the floor" technique to alleviate contraction in the low back muscles and avoid muscle cramps. Every 10 seconds, sweep the hand and knee to the floor with all motion about the hips and shoulder joints. There is no motion in the spine.

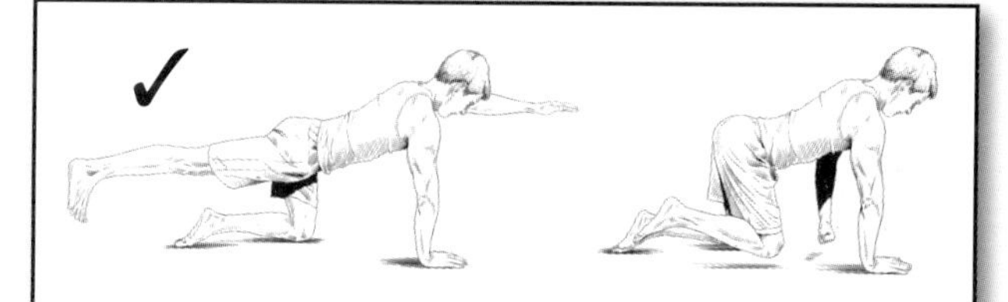

There is a tendency for some to lift the leg too high causing twist in the spine. Instead of focusing on raising the leg, "push the heel away". You will also notice more work in the back, buttock and leg muscles.

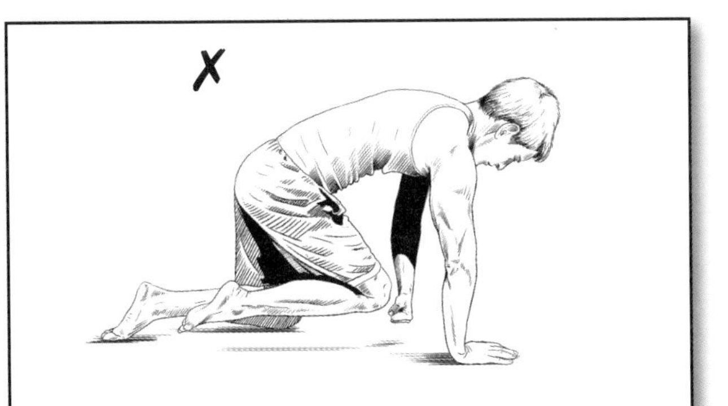

Flaws during "sweep the floor" include allowing motion to occur in the spine and neck. All motion should be in the hips and shoulders.

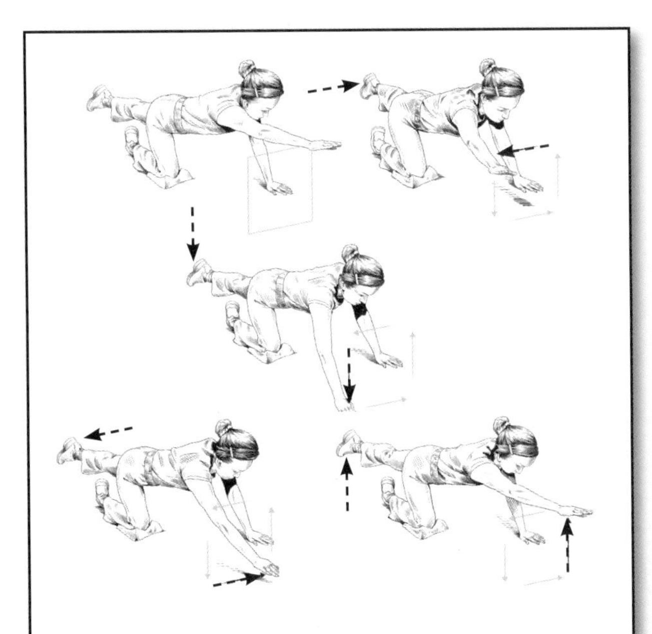

Eventually the full bird-dog is achieved. The progression continues by "drawing squares" with the hand and foot – square the hand/foot out away from the midline, down, across to the midline and up. All motion takes place about the shoulders and hips – none occurs in the spine.

The standing bird-dog for those with compromised knees

Those of you who have knees compromised with arthritis, knee replacements, or just experience difficulties getting to the floor, you may perform the bird-dog while standing. Here the same principles of core stiffness and shoulder/hip-focused motion still apply. The same 10-second holding time, and set and rep rules should be maintained as well.

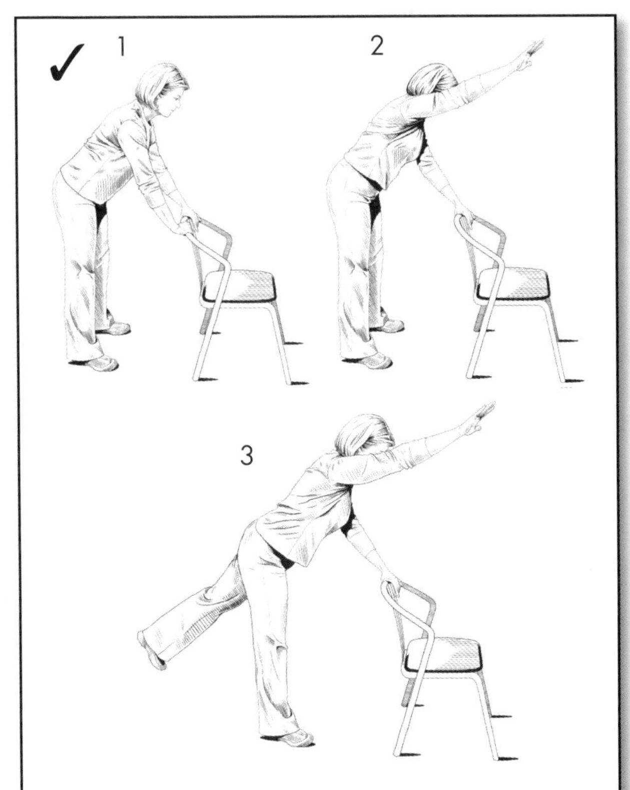

The standing bird-dog for those unable to get to the floor follows a similar progression (1). First just one arm is raised (2), then just one leg. Eventually the full bird-dog is achieved with motion only about the shoulders and hips (3).

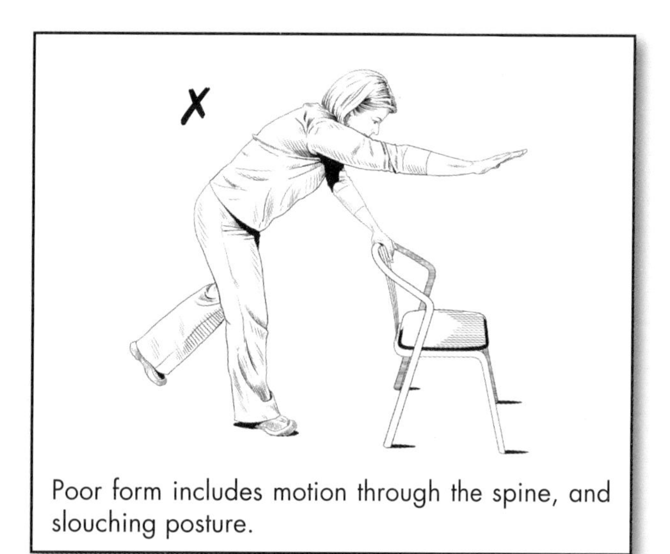

Poor form includes motion through the spine, and slouching posture.

Building Balance Around Your Back with the "Big 3"

Our research on different groups has shown that those who have balance between the big three exercises in terms of sets/reps, have a lower risk of future disorders. For example, if you perform the curlup with 6,4,2 reps, then you should perform the side bridge and bird-dog with these same numbers on both sides. You should progress these numbers equally with each of the three exercises.

When beginning the program, some of you will notice a deficit with just one exercise. Try and work towards restoring a balance where the difficulty is equal among the Big 3 when performing a balanced number of sets/reps.

Greasing the Joints: The Cat/Camel

You have now learned the non-negotiable "Big 3:" the curl-up, the side-bridge and the bird-dog. These exercises are designed to promote pain-free ability through bracing the spine into its pain-free position. All three had the common instruction to "avoid motion in the spine!" There are, however, times when people just want to move their spines. This can be healthy. We have found that the least stressful way to accomplish this is through another exercise that must be performed on all fours: the cat/camel.

The cat/camel is a gentle motion exercise. Note that this is not a stretch and therefore the end-ranges of motion (or pushing a joint to its maximum comfortable limit) are not to be pushed. It is the controlled motion that is beneficial – not any effort to stress the end-range. In fact, it is helpful for some to slightly reduce their range of motion during the exercise so that they don't feel as if they're reaching the extreme of either position.

The exercise is performed by moving smoothly back and forth from a downward spinal curve with the head looking up (the cat) to a rounded hump through the spine while the head looks down (the camel).

As with all of our exercises, our lab has measured spine stress on patients performing this activity, finding that only seven to eight cycles are needed to reduce internal spine friction or resistance to motion. Further repetitions are not necessary and may even be undoing the value of the exercise.

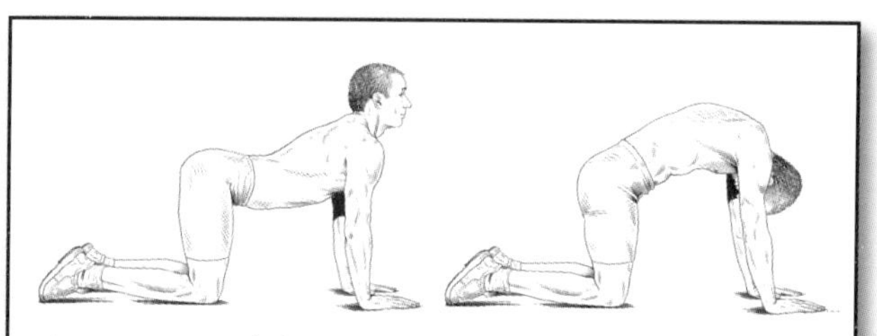

The cat-camel begins on the hands and knees. Gently flex and extend the entire spine staying within the pain-free range of motion. Each cycle should take about three to four seconds.

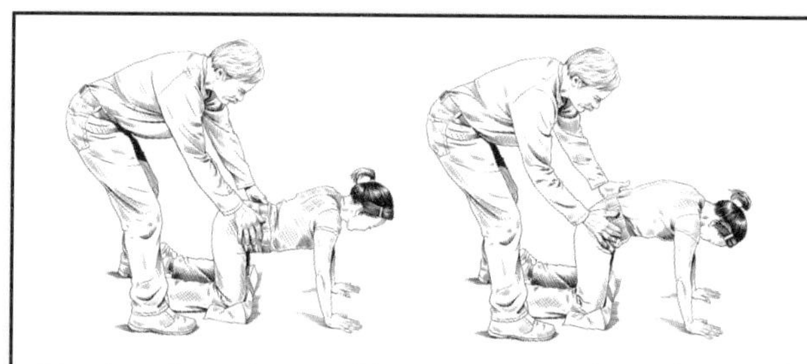

Moving the spine and hips is not easily understood by some. They will benefit from some coaching to achieve full motion from the spine and the hips.

Movement Exercises to Eliminate

No doubt you have been given some mobilizing and stretching exercises for your back. If these stretches had cured you, you wouldn't be reading this book for advice. If they do not promote the healthy spine posture and movement we've outlined so far, cut them out of your life for good! As we've previously discussed, pulling your knees to your chest should be the first thing to go! It is a quick fix and will only hurt you more long-term. And please stop lying on your back and dropping the knees to either side. These flawed positions are keeping your discs and spine joints sensitive. Do the cat/camel to give the spine some daily motion, but eliminate all other prescribed spine-motion exercises.

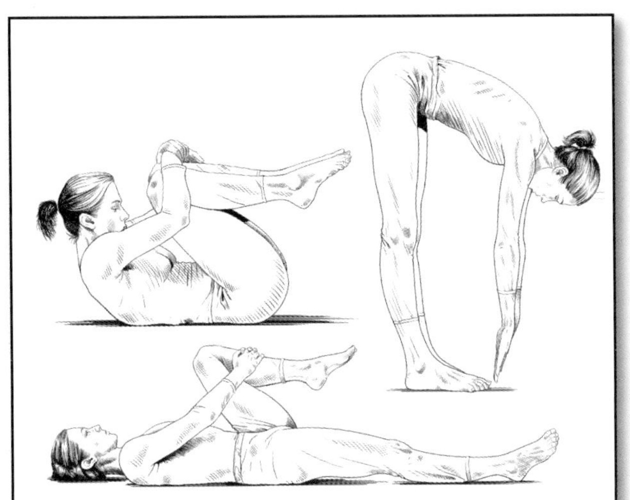

The silly stretches. Stop these and you will reduce your pain sensitivity.

The ill-advised superman: Here is another common exercise that will make a back patient worse. The "superman" is a commonly prescribed spine extensor muscle exercise that results in over 6000 N (about 1300 pounds or almost 600 kilos) of compression placed on a hyper-extended spine. It is a poorly designed exercise for people with back pain. Let's get rid of this "remedial exercise" and reserve it for those pain-free people interested in athletic gains.

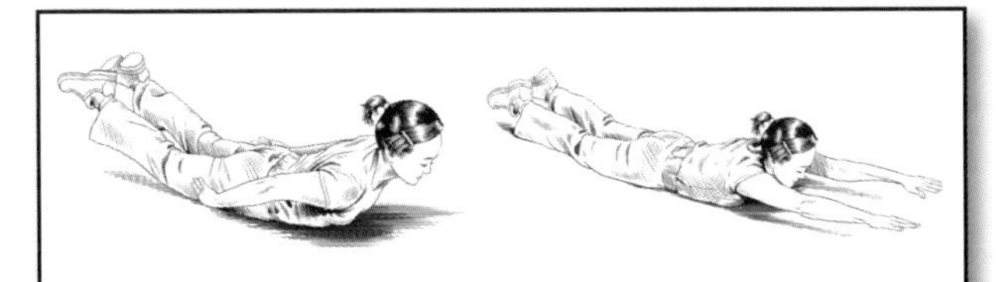

Variations of the "superman" exercise must be eliminated from the pain reduction program. Although popular in some clinics, our scientific investigations have proven they add unnecessary compressive load to the spine that is contorted into a hyper-extended posture.

Now that you have an understanding of exercise progressions to build your back from its painful state, you will need another element – walking. Once you are aware of the principles for a successful walking program we will put the core "Big 3" exercises into practice and create your program in chapter 14.

Chapter 10

The Walking Program – Nature's Back Balm

The Walking Program

Nature's Back Balm

You Can Turn Walking into a Cure

When we think of the word "balm" we think of a wax or a cream that can be applied to the body that can eliminate a number of discomforts, from chapped lips to muscle aches. We think of it as something that can be reapplied throughout the day to continue to provide comfort and relief. Although no such topical concoction exists for back pain, each of us has the capacity to apply our own sort of "back balm" through an activity that is incredibly natural but underutilized by many: walking.

Walking is one of the most commonplace and fundamental activities inherent in our daily living. While simple to do, it is extremely and uniquely important for back health. A walking program needs to be a mandatory component of your pain elimination program, plain and simple.

Scientifically speaking, with each step, the act of lifting and swinging the leg requires muscular activity to support the pelvis from sinking down on one side and bending the spine. Each step produces gentle muscle contraction, which is repeated producing the gait pattern. Very few activities challenge the lateral parts of the spine and core, and trim the hips, as well as walking. The torso becomes an energy storage system, as with each step, elastic tissues in the back reduce the muscular effort, and unload the spine. This "unloading" is further assisted with arm swing and a faster walking speed. The torso sling muscles convey the arm movements and forces into drivers for the hips. In this way, walking trains essential muscular slings that contribute to other important activities in a way that eliminates back pain.

Some of you reading this may be confused, as you have found walking to increase your pain. You may have previously been given poor advice. It is likely you were told that walking slowly and leisurely would reduce your pain, but in doing just that you haven't experienced any relief. This is usually because walking too slowly actually statically loads the spine. The muscles add more crushing forces to the spine. On top of that, poor posture while walking will only worsen the pain. So our plan is to first correct the walking posture to reduce strain on the painful parts, and then create a healthy walking pattern to eliminate pain.

In contrast to slow walking or "mall strolling", moving more briskly usually changes walking from a cause of pain to a pain reliever. If you find that even a quickly paced walk hurts, either your pain sensitivity must be particularly high at this point in your recovery, or you are trying to walk too far in one session. This simply means that you may have to wait until you are further along before you add this component into your routine. In the meantime, follow the process outlined in the previous chapters, and eventually you will obtain relief with faster walking.

Other negative issues with the slow walk include the tendency to not swing your arms, further adding to the static muscle cramp. It is also common to lock the knee in full extension with each step. This removes the spring action of the leg muscles needed for pain-free walking.

We've established that a faster pace is crucial, but other postural components are equally as important in perfecting a therapeutic walk. Pavel Tsatsouline, the Russian strongman makes interesting distinctions between cultural groups and how they walk. He claims that Americans generally look down at the ground while walking causing them to lead with their head cocked forwards. In contrast, Russians generally lead with their chest. This naturally promotes arm swing. This is the goal!

Walking with a Pain-Free Style

Observe your walking style in front of a mirror, a shop front window or have a friend take a video of you on their smart phone. Are you chin-poking, walking without swinging the arms or taking small steps? Are you looking down like the American? Or do you have a puffed out walk like the Russian? Be aware of your current style, then try the following corrections (see pics):

1. Achieve the corrected upright standing posture you have found to relieve pain. This will also prevent back muscle cramping.

2. Lightly stiffen the abdominal muscles.
3. Try a few marching steps. This means moving strongly and deliberately but in one place, lifting the knees slightly higher than you usually would.
4. Begin walking, swinging the arms about the shoulders - not the elbows. Recall the walking figure in Chapter 8.
5. Progress with larger and faster steps, until you establish a walk that "means business." Move like you have somewhere to be.

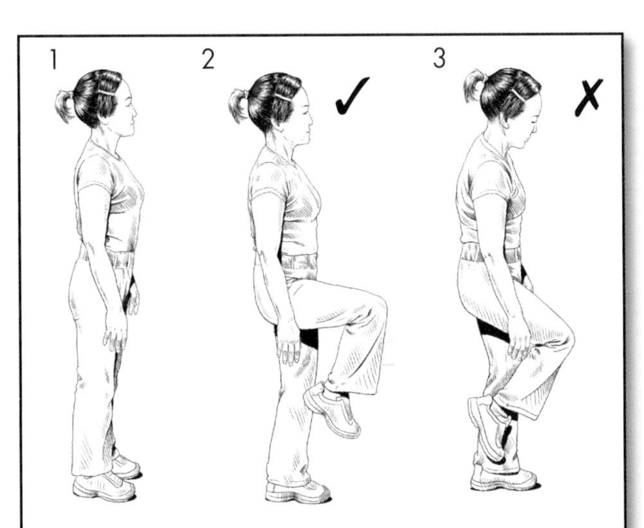

(1) First stand "tall" using corrections from previous chapters. (2) The ability to stand, balance and walk begins with standing on one leg. Begin standing upright. Stiffen the torso and raise one leg only using hip motion. No spine motion occurs. (3) Poor form consists of spine motion, poor balance, dropping the hip on the leg raise side, allowing the hip to shift laterally. Corrective strategies include gripping the floor with the foot, stiffening the torso more.

How to Build a Pain-Free Walking Program

Some of you with high pain sensitivity will need to begin the walking program with short bursts performed on a frequent basis. If, for example, you experience pain after walking say ten steps, the logical rehab protocol is to take six to eight steps every hour on the hour. You do not have the pain-free ability at the present time to train with a professional – you will break into pain with every activity. Your goal is to work on your own to increase your ability to move without pain, and increase the volume of work you are able to perform pain-free.

This is the rationale behind interval training: training sessions are organized to slowly and methodically increase tolerance to pain. Through hourly walks, you will gain the number of steps that can be taken pain-free. As you continue to progress, the time between training sessions is also increased. Slowly, and methodically, you will reach the ultimate goal, which is to walk for half an hour three times per day – before breakfast, around midday and after dinner.

During this period in which you are continuing to lengthen your walks, you will likely benefit from taking "micro-breaks". A micro-break essentially involves pausing in the middle of your walk to rest and check in with your posture. The truth is, people often lose their walking "good form" as they fatigue. If pain is impending, stop walking. Perform the drill to realign the lumbar spine and hips into the pain-free posture you learned in chapter 8. Clinicians call it "elastic equilibrium", you call it your "sweet spot" position. This can be done at a park bench, perhaps stopping to briefly chat with someone. Now resume walking, enjoying the relief! We will further discuss this spine-sparing concept when looking at stenosis-specific recovery in chapter 14.

Once successful here you will graduate to enjoying longer walks. At this point, not only will you have attained success in increasing your walking mobility but you will also find that your abilities to perform other enjoyable activities have increased as well!

Progressing the Walking Program

Once you have found success with the daily walking prescription of 30 minutes three times per day, try a longer walk. Make note of how you feel the next day, as your body will be telling you whether or not you are ready for this step. Once you have experienced several pain-free weeks that include some longer walks, you may want to try a slow, short jog. If this feels good, repeat your jog for the next three days, after which you must take five days off. You may continue your walks, but rest from the jogs. It is noteworthy at this point to state that jogging is not necessary for back health, I simply mention it for those wishing to resume this activity if it is their goal. The trick is to stimulate the tissues to heal and gristle while not allowing the cumulative trauma to get ahead of the healing. If you want to work jogging into your schedule more permanently, take a week off every two to three weeks. This is the key to long term success.

Walking up or down an incline can be your friend or foe. Progressions for walking should eventually include walking up hill, on a gradual slope to begin with. Then try walking backwards uphill, with mindful focus on extending and pushing with the knees. Try lifting your arms overhead to foster a more upright, backwards walking posture. You will experience the leg training and know that you have done some good work.

As you can see, walking, like any other exercise for a back patient must begin slowly and build up to a more challenging level day by day. Pushing yourself to a point where you begin to experience pain is not a sign you need to drive through it, but rather that you need to stop, and build a smaller set of daily goals for yourself tomorrow. Yes, it takes patience, but good things come to those who wait.

Chapter 11
The Core Program

The Core Program

Now you have the skills and guidance to create your daily program. This will be sufficient for many who simply want to enjoy daily life without pain and maintain modest capabilities. Work these into your schedule each day and you will reap the benefits.

Remember no exercise program will help if poor movement habits prevail throughout the day. Thus all day long, remove the cause with spine hygiene, including the movement tools adapted to all movements.

The reasonably active individual will begin gently with the remedial exercises found in the "Big 3" chapter. Try a few repetitions and wait until the next day to see if your body found them tolerable. Slowly add repetitions to your sessions each week as long as you are improving. For those with low tolerance and the tendency to break into pain during low levels of exercise, recall the approach to have several sessions throughout the day of just a few repetitions. The more robust individual will be able to have a more rigorous session perhaps once per day. Repetitions are added to each exercise as your sessions progress.

Here is a guideline of what a typical person would achieve after about four to six weeks:

1. **Cat-camel:** eight slow repetitions, rest, perform another eight reps.
2. **Bird-dog:** six reps of 10 seconds holding the right arm and left leg in extension then sweeping the floor in between each hold. Repeat with the other arm-leg. Rest 30 seconds. For the next set, reduce your number of reps by two. Therefore perform four reps on the right and four on the left. Rest. Then two reps on each side. Finish.
3. **Curl-up:** six reps of 10-second holds. Rest 30 seconds. Four reps. Rest. Two reps. Finish.
4. **Side-Bridge:** six reps of 10-second holds on the right, and six reps on the left. Rest 30 seconds. Then four reps on each side. Rest. Two reps on each side. Finish.
5. **Walking:** 30 minutes walking before work, 20 minutes at lunch and 30 minutes after dinner.

Do not be concerned if you recover more slowly. But you should have a positive slope in symptom reduction. Use the workbook in the appendix to assist in creating and documenting your program. This will help guide your progression or exercise regression to ensure symptom reduction.

When you feel that more challenge is needed, add one repetition to each set, do not add to the 10 second holding time. This strategy will reduce cramps in the back muscles and build endurance. Never sacrifice good exercise form to accomplish more repetitions.

As the program continues to develop you will naturally experience increased hip mobilization. Many report that they sleep better without pain during the night. Keep the disciplined approach to spine hygiene. Enjoy pain-free living again. Prepare to explain to your friends, family and colleagues how you became your own back mechanic and cured your back pain! They'll all be curious to learn your secret for looking, acting and moving so differently.

There it is – the program that has helped thousands regain a pain-free back. There will be a few of you who need more work. You have special, and more rare conditions that will need some additional work. In addition there will be those wanting higher than average pain-free capacity. These individuals should read on.

Chapter 12

Restoring the Hips

Restoring the Hips

Back pain, and hip pain, inhibit the gluteal muscles resulting in more back and hip pain. However, trying to address hip deficiencies too early when back pain is still present leads to frustration and more grief. **I repeat, do not stretch your hamstrings or hips early in the program. Let the pain sensitivity cool down.** When your back pain has settled, and you have gained some load and motion resilience, you may try to restore your hips. This involves mobilizing the hips to enhance controlled motion, together with re-establishing healthy activation patterns.

Mobilize the Hips

Stiff hips result in more motion transferred to the spine, and this is a feature we are trying to avoid. In those with hip arthritis, enhancing mobility in them will be tricky without flaring them into pain. But in others, you may follow the following protocol. Also, remember that achievable hip mobility is governed by your anatomy. You may or may not get as much mobility as your colleagues but that is ok. A competent clinician can assess the source of hip stiffness and guide you on this. They will be able to inform you of the range of motion and source of stiffness as to whether it is due to the hip joint capsule, the shape of the acetabulum (socket), tight and sensitive nerves, or the muscles. Many of these cannot be stretched to reduce pain sensitivity and enhance motion. The "hip airplane" is a wonderful mobilizing drill (do not treat it as a stretch).

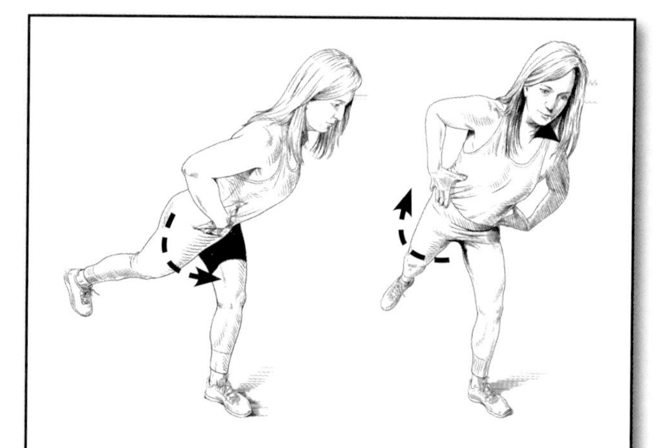

The "hip airplane" is an advanced hip mobilization tactic that uses a fundamental movement pattern – hip external rotation. The hip airplane works wonders for enhancing hip mobility and for those with back pain but rarely hip pain. Use your thumb on the ribs and fingers on the iliac crest of the pelvic ring as cues to ensure there is no spine motion – all motion is about the hip joint. Use the foot grip tactic learned during squatting to enhance balance.

While back pain inhibits the gluteal muscles of the hip it also tends to facilitate, or tighten, the psoas muscle crossing the front of the hip coursing up the side of the spine. First, let's address the consequence of back pain on the psoas. If you have had symptoms of a lax pelvic ring, this may have been caused by performing excessive numbers of lunges—avoid lunges as these exercises are not for you given your history.

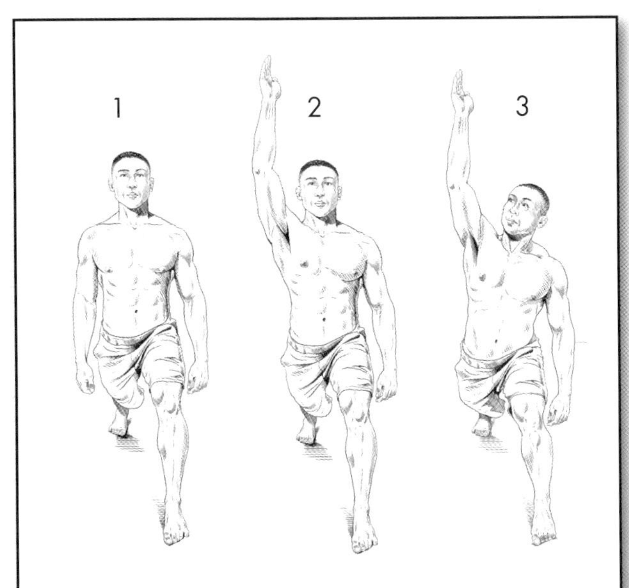

The lunge mobilizes the hips. Adopt a lunge position (1). Push the hand overhead on the same side as the extended hip, as you descend into the lunge (2). Bend the torso slightly away from the extended hip and drop the shoulder back to further target and stretch the psoas (3). Complete the exercise by taking a walking stride switching legs and the raised arm. This is the "walking lunge". The goal is to lunge-walk for six strides.

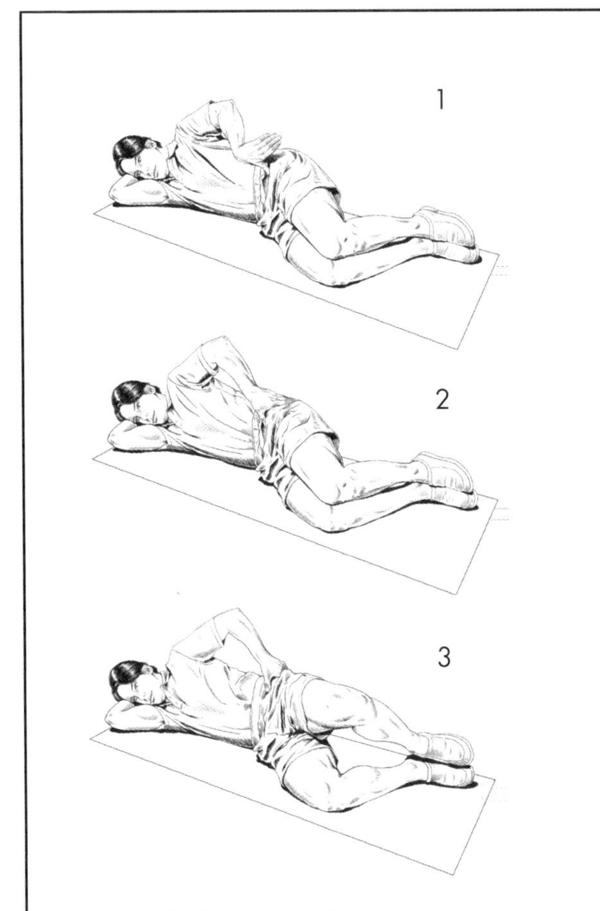

The clamshell exercise begins with the thumb placed on the Anterior-superior-iliac-spine of the pelvis (the bony lump on the iliac crests lateral to the navel) (1). This targets the fingers to the gluteus medius (2). Now as you open the knees like a clam you will feel the gluteal muscle contract (3). Focus your mind on this contraction and skillfully master the ability to contract it at will. Do not allow the spine to twist.

Recall that back pain often leaves a legacy of inhibition of the gluteal muscles. Now we can reintegrate the gluteal muscles back into your movement patterns. The most effective exercises we have documented to achieve this are clamshell exercises and back bridges – but you must pay attention to the technique.

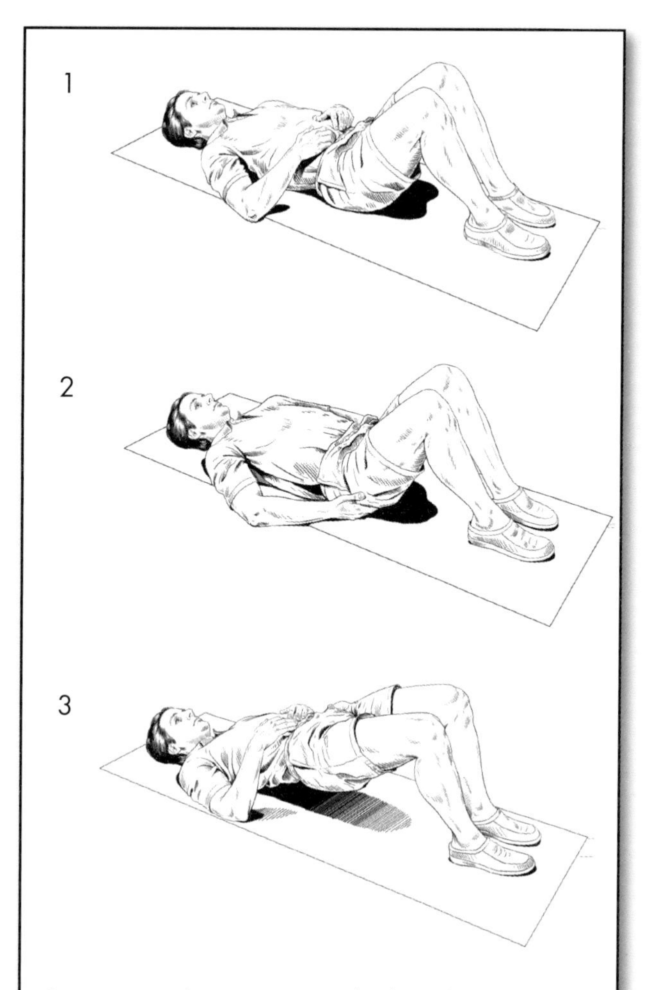

Once you have mastered the clamshell you are ready for the back bridge. First learn to just contract gluteus maximus by clenching your buttocks. (1) There must be no motion observable particularly in the spine. You may feel the muscles contract. (2) Then by mindfully focussing on the gluteus maximus contraction, and only using this contraction, intensify the gluteus squeeze causing the pelvis to raise. There should be no hamstring muscle contraction (3). You may need coaching to achieve this – ask your therapist to follow our DVD on therapeutic exercise and follow the coaching cues.

Some readers want to advance further. While outside of the scope of this book, I show more hip progressions to address this issue in "*Ultimate Back Fitness and Performance*".

Pain originating from the hips themselves requires a much more sophisticated approach and is outside of the scope of this book. See a good clinician. But briefly, when moving the hip joint into positions close to its current end-range of motion, gentle joint traction can be applied with great success. Gentle traction can, in the hands of a skilled clinician, extend the hip-joint range-of-motion.

Preserving the Deep Squat Ability and Hip Mobility

You will hear people state that children have the ability to deep squat and that it is dysfunctional that adults lose this ability. This rationale is used to justify performing deep squats with barbells and dumbbells. This is problematic on several levels, particularly for those with back pain. Children are not mini adults. They have disproportionally shorter legs. It is to their mechanical advantage to squat with what is considered good form very deeply. When in the womb, their hips and knees are bent into a squat posture. But as they develop into adults their hip sockets deepen to provide stability for load bearing when upright. This causes a collision of the thigh bone (femur) and the anterior hip socket (acetabulum and labrum). Some of you with hip pain will have been diagnosed with anterior femoral impingement – perhaps from following the instruction to squat deeply. There is no evidence to support that squatting deeply with a barbell under tutelage from your personal trainer will preserve the ability to squat any better than body weight. Wisdom from several non-western cultures suggests that simply squatting under body weight once per day will preserve the squat ability. Furthermore, for those with back pain and hip pain, squatting this way just once will not flare up the painful condition.

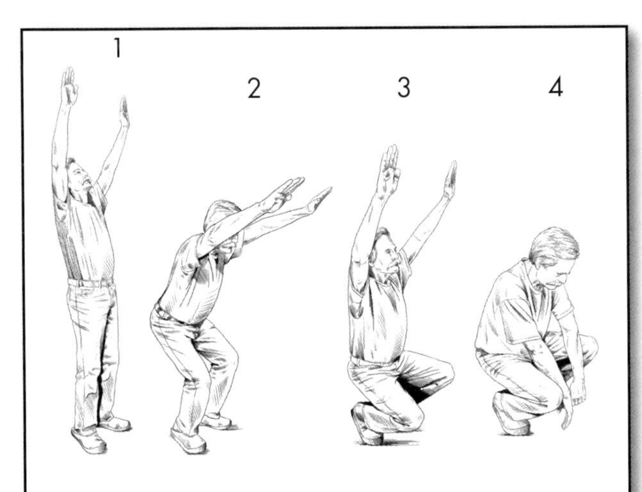

To preserve squatting ability do this drill once per day: Reach overhead extending your spine (1), and hip hinge to descend (2). Slowly approach the deep squat (3), and then take the tension out by lowering the arms and relaxing for a few moments (4). To ascend, reverse the process.

HERE IS HOW TO EXECUTE THE BODY WEIGHT SQUAT:

1. Stand with your feet wide enough to find the most shallow part of your hip socket (these tests are in *Low Back Disorders*).
2. Squat down trying to maintain the neutral spine curves.
3. Settle into the bottom of the squat and try to completely relax. Remove all tension from the legs, hips and pelvis.
4. Then build tension, and rise out of the squat moving the hips back and into the short-stop, then finish by pulling the hips through as you stand upright.
5. Do not repeat. One repetition is enough.

Chapter 13

Next Level Training: Regaining Your Active Lifestyle

Next Level Training

Regaining Your Active Lifestyle

It's time to examine the steps towards a more complete recovery in terms of regaining your fitness. Some of you will be satisfied with what we have achieved so far as you have reduced your pain. Continue exercising with the "Big 3" and practicing spine hygiene everyday. Keep in mind however, that you are not invincible. You have a chance of relapsing if you return to your former movement patterns and stop the daily exercise routine, so maintain the discipline and keep doing what you're doing. If you're happy where you are, you should skip the rest of this chapter.

For others, you may miss playing pick-up basketball with your kids, dancing with your spouse or cycling with your friends. If you are serious about enhancing your athletic ability, I will direct you to my previous book entitled *"Ultimate Back Fitness and Performance"*. But for now, this chapter offers you a brief introduction to enhancing strength and injury resilience within patterns of movement. Remember: keep your movement pristine, and never compromise good form to increase or prolong your performance.

Resistance Exercise

Strengthening for performance and injury resilience means adhering to a resistance training regimen. Resistance training, when done correctly, can be beneficial for former pain sufferers – technique is key. Unfortunately, many patients are given the wrong resistance exercises, shown faulty techniques and asked to adhere to cookie-cutter rehab regimens that do not take into account the unique aspect of their personal history.

Not all progressive resistance exercises are created equal. I've proven this time and again in our published research papers. For example, any type of weighted single arm cable pull, creates twisting forces that impose inordinate loads on your spine. Because of the way that muscles work to support twist, there is much more load on the spine than in those tasks where forces are side to side (frontal plane), or forward and backward such as when doing a pushup. Always begin with exercises that create resistance forward and backward in the sagittal plane. Then, if tolerated well, add frontal exercises and finally, if tolerated add "stop-twist" challenges. Note that the spine is not twisted – the exercises impose twisting forces but the goal is to prevent twisting and keep the spine in a neutral position.

Adding Resistance

In an ideal world, resistance training involves choosing the right resistance load. Unfortunately, those capable of prescribing the right resistance exercise to those with a back pain history, and who are able to demonstrate the required precise techniques are rare individuals indeed. Remember that you are often your own best guide. Always adhere to these key principles:

- Never sacrifice exercise form to lift or move more load.
- Only add more load when your spine is in a neutral posture that is possible to maintain.

Divide Training into Movement Patterns, not Targeted Body Parts

The concept of resistance training has been hijacked by bodybuilders and by those with the sole goal of training for appearance's sake. Following their advice will likely erase your progress and take you right back to a place of daily pain. Forget those "workouts" where you aim to train the biceps, pectorals or legs in isolation. Replace them with precise patterns of movement, and exercises that enhance your ability to move in joint sparing but competent ways. The four main resistance categories you should focus on are Pushes, Pulls, Lifts and Carries. More on these later.

Patient Files: A recent example came in a consult with a former world champion powerlifter who could not even bend over without pain – this in a man who has squatted holding nearly half a ton! Within 15 minutes into the session he had re-discovered how corrected movement patterns with the right amount of muscle stiffness in his torso restored pain-free lifting of 200 pounds from the floor. It was "in him" all of the time but pain had altered his movement and muscle activation patterns.

Patterns for Strength, Endurance and Power Development

Athleticism wins competition. That being said, heightened fitness should never be reserved for those looking to get a gold medal at the Olympics. The same athleticism allows a plumber to get through a hard, productive day at work without pain, or a busy mom to multitask, running around the house to finish the laundry and get the kids dressed before soccer practice at 6:30 pm. For our purposes, athleticism stems from being able to push and pull with gusto but no pain. It stems from the ability to lift, sparing the joints and harnessing hip power. It is displayed during forceful effort requiring the stop-twist pattern, such as opening a large heavy door, as the forces are directed through the body linkage in a way to never cause pain. Athleticism is the foundation for carrying loads, walking, running, turning and cutting, lunging and returning to position. It is used to restore balance during a slip to react quickly and appropriately to arrest the fall. You get the idea. Here are some thoughts for training in movement patterns to increase your athleticism together with some hip specific patterns. Build sets and reps following the familiar descending pyramid shown in chapter 11.

At this point you should be relatively pain-free during everyday activity. I will introduce a simple push and a pull exercise to add to your routine. Try just adding these two for now. Again, progressions for all of the other patterns are well addressed in my book *"Ultimate Back Fitness and Performance"*.

Push Exercises

Many core exercises fall into the push category. The "stir the pot" exercise trains the entire "front side" of the body known as the anterior chain. Push-ups are another fantastic challenge for the entire anterior chain. There are many ways to modify the classic push-up in order to better integrate the hips.

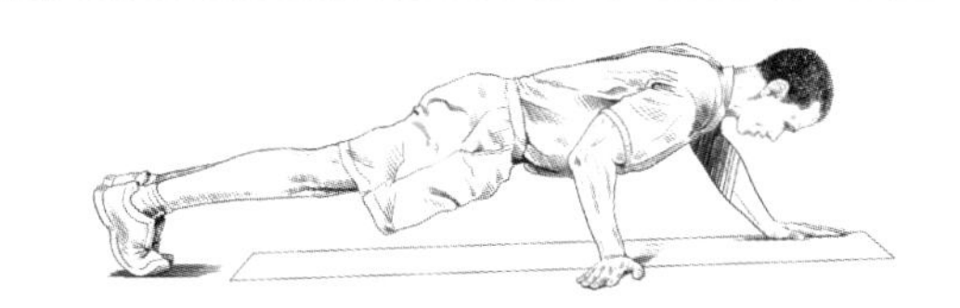

A superior stabilizing push-up. Note the form that must be strictly maintained – the body is aligned without the spine slumping into extension or the hips hiking up into flexion.

While the exercise may begin with the hands aligned normally, the progression continues with "staggered hands" meaning one extends to the side, and the other above the vertical line from the shoulder. This adds challenge to maintain the perfect alignment of the torso. Allowing the body to bend constitutes poor form.

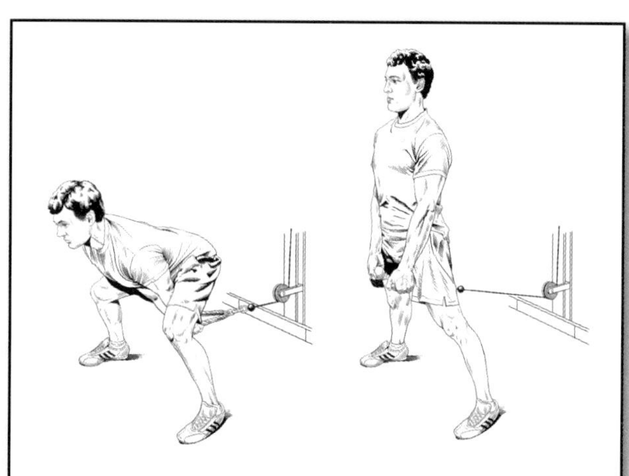

The cable pull is a different style of push exercise that integrates the hip hinge with a stiffened core to assist with lifting and moving large objects. Try loading 20 pounds onto the cable machine with the block set in its lowest position. Try 8 repetitions with perfect form, then 6 for set 2, then 4 for set 3. If perfect form was maintained, you may increase the load.

Pull Exercises

Push exercises should be balanced with pulls – for each push, try and complete one pull. Pull-ups are an ideal counter exercise for push-ups because they challenge the posterior chain – the muscles down the back. An excellent way to begin pulls is to use suspension straps that are made by several manufacturers.

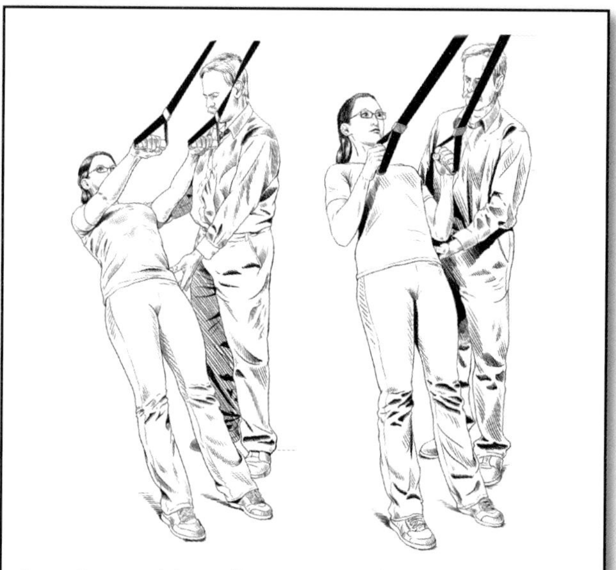

Standing cable pulls require a lot of setup. Grab the handles with the arms pronated (palms down) and squeeze harder than necessary. Squeeze the gluteal muscles. Pull the shoulder blades together and downwards using latissimus dorsi. Ensure the spine posture is maintaining the neutral curves. Use this discipline to ensure that there is no way pain can enter your back. Now pull with the arms with motion only occurring at the arms/shoulders. Eliminate even the smallest spine movement. Stiffen your whole body putting more "effort" into the pull than is actually necessary. Notice as the pull occurs, the hands are rotated into a hammer grip as they approach the chest to create minimal loading on the shoulder and elbow joints. Use the same set/rep numbers as in the push exercise.

In today's society, many have lost athleticism in their hands. Too much time is spent computing and what resistance work is done involves gripping small handles. Controlling objects with strong hands will ultimately spare the back. To combat this trend and balance the ability to grip and control objects, we usually begin hose or rope pulling progressions. This is also an excellent start on training aerobic conditioning.

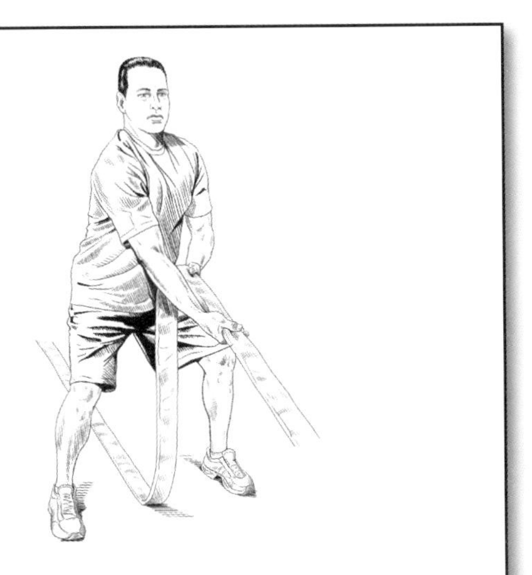

Fire hose pulls or rope pulls involve hand-over-hand pulling. Good form requires sitting back as if in a chair. Neutral spine curves are maintained. Of particular importance here is to avoid the torso from twisting – instead the pelvis is swivelled around the hip joints sparing the spine. The hose is pulled directly into the navel with short chops – do not get greedy taking in too much hose as this causes spine twist. This is an excellent start on aerobic conditioning.

Section in Conclusion

There you have it - a few exercises to help enhance your athletic ability and get you closer to participating in the activities you love. With practice, commitment and adherence to proper form, you'll gain strength, resilience and resistance to injury.

Again, the section within this book on advanced exercise is purposefully brief. Creating the right progressions to guarantee your success in regaining athletic ability, when one has a history of back pain, requires expertise. Risking repetition I advise the reader to refer to my textbook *"Ultimate Back Fitness and Performance"* (www.backfitpro.com) for a much more comprehensive guide to enhancing athleticism while successfully managing a history of back pain.

Part 4:
Fine Tuning the Machine for Best Performance

Chapter 14

Considerations for Special Conditions: Sciatica, Kyphosis, Scoliosis, Stenosis, the Overweight and Others

Considerations for Special Conditions

Sciatica, Kyphosis, Scoliosis, Stenosis, the Overweight and Others

Some of you, prior to reading this book, had been given specific diagnoses for your pain by a doctor. At this stage in your reading, your self-assessment should be able to confirm or deny your physician's diagnosis. As we've previously discussed, having a label for your back condition is often not as helpful as being able to identify the movements, postures and loads that are your pain triggers. That being said, there are some special considerations to be taken into account when recovering from certain "labelled" conditions. Here are some approaches that often help if you fall into one of these unique categories of back pain. I remind you once again that your primary health care physician is not likely familiar with the approaches in this book, so please show them my suggestions. Make sure that there are no other existing medical conditions preventing you from participating in these exercises and recommendations.

Sciatica

Sciatica refers to pain experienced anywhere along the length of the sciatic nerve. This nerve travels, from the lowest two lumbar joints, through the buttock region and behind the hip joints, down the back of the thigh, the front and side of the shin and finally to the foot and toes.

Interestingly, if you experience sciatica-related toe pain you will be able to identify the location along the nerve route that is troublesome. Pain in the big toe indicates irritation of the fifth lumbar root (L5) while irritation in the four little toes indicates the fourth lumbar root (L4). I have had patients with terrible foot pain, even to the point where a doctor suggested foot amputation. Their pains were purely from a pinched sciatic nerve in the lumbar spine. The truth is, that even though the pain could be experienced anywhere along this route, its origins can be traced back to a pinch, or compression, in the lumbar spine.

The nerve irritation has a variety of possible causes. The pinch may be related to bulged disc material, or from arthritic bone, or ligaments thickened from arthritis, or joint capsules that are a legacy of injury and overuse. Sorting these out during a competent clinical exam is important as it helps refine the treatment.

As with all successful treatment, ***the key is to remove the cause and not merely treat the symptoms***. If disc material is the suspected culprit, try the postures that you discovered in the assessment chapter to reduce and eliminate pain. Practicing good spine hygiene is often successful in shrinking the offending disc material that is responsible for irritating the nerve. Any leg pain will typically increase with periods of prolonged sitting so practice varying postures. It is also problematic to lift heavy objects, as this will further irritate the already sensitive nerve. Typically, the pain caused by sciatica can be relieved through walking using tolerable intervals. Essentially, avoid prolonged sitting, repeated spinal flexing and stretching. Stretching a painful sciatic nerve will only make it more sensitive. Yet, ***many mistakenly think stretching their hamstring muscles is the solution***.

Another cause for chronic sciatica is the arthritic changes that occur as we age. Bones continue to grow even as we get older, and as they expand they compromise the normal space reserved for the nerve root. For this type of sciatica, pain is usually aggravated by exercise (sometimes even walking), and seemingly innocent postures like lying on the back in a sagging bed that takes the back out of its natural curve. ***The key is to reestablish and maintain your "neutral postures."*** I often use "modified walking" as therapy in my consults with patients—I insist on proper walking technique based on pain-free intervals that we introduced in chapter 10. We turn painful walking into the therapy. Begin by finding a posture to reduce the radiating symptoms such as lying quietly on the tummy for a few minutes. Then walk until the radiating symptoms just begin. Now you will need to restore your spine to a pain-free state. Try "wall-walking", or decompressing the spine on a park bench. Once the pain is reduced, try another bout of walking and repeat the cycle. This technique often helps reduce sciatic symptoms and restore pain-free fitness.

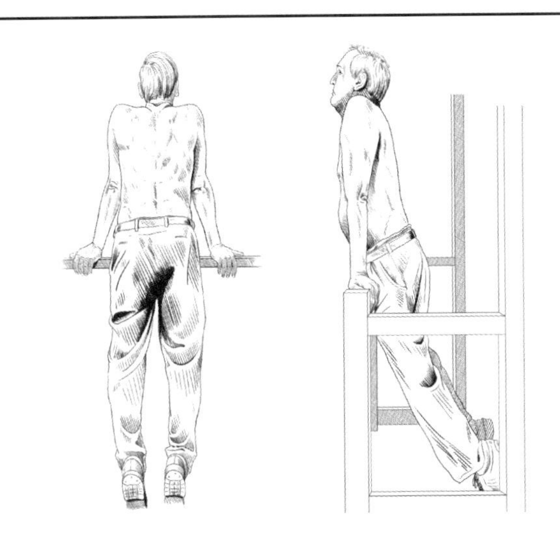

"Park bench" decompression. Walking begins, and just as discomfort starts you move to a strategically placed park bench, or a strong railing, where you can perform this posture at regular intervals. Push the "heels" of the hands down while posting your bodyweight up over your arms. Keeping your arms hugged tight to your torso, carry your weight down your arms. Then try and work the hips towards the bar to extend the spine. This decompressing posture is held as long as it is comfortable but no longer than a minute. Ideally, symptoms are lessened or eliminated at this point. Now repeat the walk until the next cycle of pain. Repeat the training session each day slowly adding more intervals. This technique aids in achieving pain-free walking through cumulative intervals.

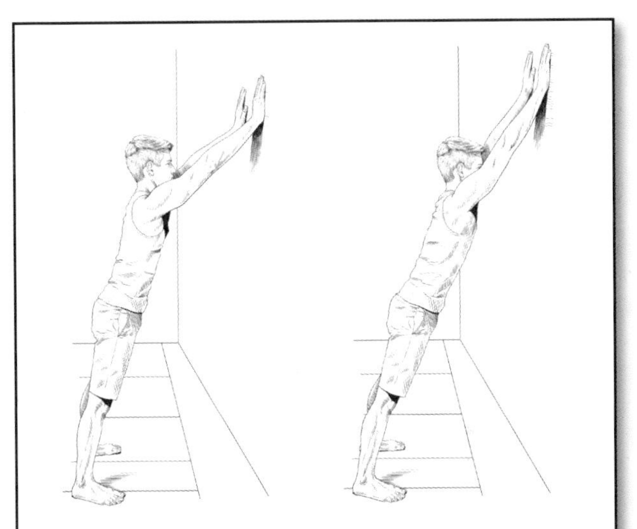

Wall walking. Another restorative technique known as arm walking or wall walking starts with you placing one hand above the other literally walking your hands up the wall. Coaching the hips to move toward the wall helps to achieve the desired upright posture.

In contrast to standard stretching, when dealing with sciatica, we will consider moving the nerves without stretching or tensioning them. This will reduce their pain sensitivity. A pinch reduces their ability to slide and move. Your objective is use non-irritating movement patterns to facilitate their continual sliding ability. In this sense, the beneficial "sliding" of the sciatic nerve to treat sciatica is opposite to tendonitis treatment in which more movement increases inflammation causing even more restriction on the tendons. This is the fundamental foundation for a term we have coined "nerve flossing". Flossing between teeth removes debris and creates more room between them. The floss moves freely with less friction when working on clean teeth. While the mechanisms are slightly different, in effect "nerve flossing" the sciatic nerve through the body's canals reduces irritation and pain sensitivity. As the nerve continues to move with increasingly less friction, the threshold for pain increases, allowing more activities to be pain-free. Nerve flossing has helped many to reduce and eliminate the painful "radiating" sensations down the buttocks and/or legs that are associated with sciatica.

Nerve Flossing Exercises

Your goal is to train and exercise and move in ways that encourage the nerves to "slide," without tensing them and causing further irritation. Contrary to stretching, this tactic will settle the nerves down. The object is to pull the nerve from one end while releasing from the other. Then reverse the process with each cycle of movement.

> **TICKLING THE DRAGON'S TAIL**
>
> Caution: You are essentially tickling the dragon's tail and there is a chance that you could get burned and the symptoms worsen. Flossing can both cure and cause pain. Try flossing 10 reps per side on the first day. See how you feel the next day. If the radiating symptoms are worse, then stop immediately. In a week, try again. However, this time try lying on your tummy first for about three minutes following the technique explained shortly. If you have the same pain increase, then this approach is not for you. On the other hand, if your symptoms have not changed, or have improved, continue with flossing. Flossing can desensitize a nerve over time and you can begin to experience relief anywhere from within a few days to a couple of months.

The technique: To begin the technique, try sitting on a desk where you can swing your legs underneath you without touching the floor. Extend your neck to look up while extending one of your knees straight in front of you, flexing the foot and toes skyward. This is performed as a smooth movement. Repeat the movement in the opposite direction: the neck is flexed; the knee, ankle, and toes are also flexed. The entire cycle (one back and forth) should take about three to four seconds. The movement of the neck and leg should be coordinated. A helpful visual is to imagine the sciatic nerve as a single cord running from the crown of your head through to the ends of your toes. By manipulating these end points back and forth you are gently moving the nerve through its canals and naturally relieving its tension.

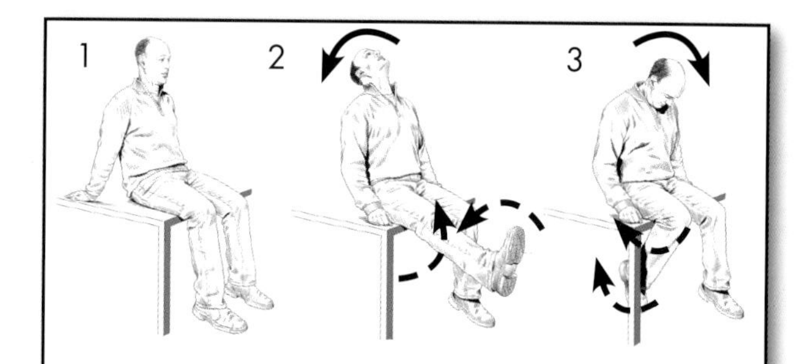

Nerve flossing technique. Find a pain free sitting posture, opening the hips and achieving a neutral spine. Sit on something with enough room to swing the leg freely (1). To floss the irritated nerve roots, extend the knee and neck at the same time creating a fluid and coordinated movement. Also dorsi-flex the ankle (pull the foot up) (2). Then perform the opposite motion as the neck and knee are flexed and the foot is plantar-flexed in a co-ordinated fashion (3). Repeat this cycle 10 times per leg.

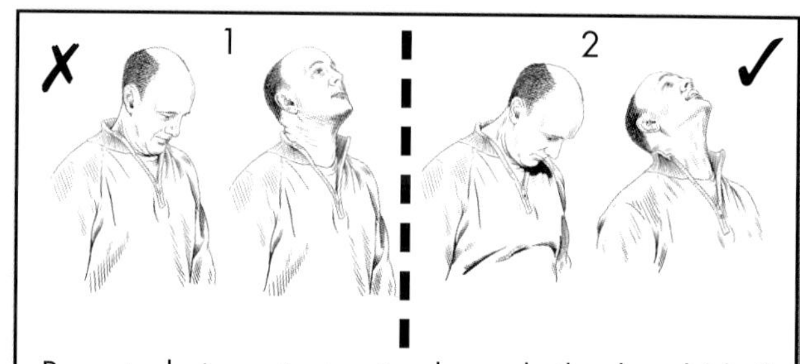

Poor technique is to simply rock the head/skull on the neck (1) which does little to alter tension in the nerve roots. Optimal technique is to flex and extend the neck (2).

Fine Details: For some, a mere three to four days of performing flossing exercises will settle and reduce radiating sciatic pains. For others, the full positive effects may take several weeks. Here are a few tips that can enhance the efficacy of nerve flossing: first and foremost, work to reduce whatever is irritating the nerve root! For example, if you can determine that the source of the pain is due to a disc bulge, then adopt a posture to reduce the size of the bulge prior to flossing. The best way to prepare the back posture for nerve flossing is to perform the relief exercise in which you lie on your stomach supporting your chin with your fists for three minutes. If you find that this helps relieve your sciatic symptoms, perform this exercise prior to flossing. If your symptoms are at their worst first thing in the morning after rising from bed, floss later in the day. If they are at their worst later in the day, floss earlier.

Stenosis

Although we've already briefly covered stenosis, let's take a closer look at this common condition. As many people age, particularly those who lived lifestyles characterized by lots of spine motion (plumbers, recreational soccer and squash players, etc.) they tend to develop arthritic changes in the vertebrae. This process of bone growth narrows the canals through which the spinal cord and nerve roots travel. The resulting condition is called stenosis, meaning "narrowing". Those with stenosis lose the ability to walk longer distances without back and leg pain. Their activity level continues to decline, and their general health follows.

Another cause of "stenosis symptoms" is vascular congestion and backup of spine fluid alongside the nerves. If this is the pain trigger, bending forward can increase the canal size and re-establish blood flow and reduce congestion. Pelvic tilting to add slight flexion to the spine can be relieving for standing and walking. Nerve flossing can assist. Core exercises particularly for the anterior abdominal muscles may also assist. But experiment to find what helps and hurts – only you will know.

Many stenosis sufferers find relief with brief bouts of traction force. In other words, **the "pulling" of the spine from one end to the other in an act of decompression can be beneficial to stenosis sufferers.** In fact, this is the only group of back patients in which traction therapy has been shown to be broadly effective.

Typically, a stenosis patient would be able to walk for a few minutes before their pain symptoms set in. Longer duration standing and walking usually causes pain and/or weakness. Many therapists teach these patients how to stay in spine flexion. We have very good success with those who have failed this approach by doing the opposite. More flexion in daily activity is often counterproductive as the posture results in more spine loading, not less. You see why the stenosis patient is often confused as to what approach to follow. We give them spine extension drills and the corrective interval walking program to add to the non-negotiable "Big 3" and spine hygiene approaches.

Restoring and preserving the ability to walk with minimal symptoms is of utmost importance. Try the same technique as we described in the earlier sciatica section of walking in a park with benches. Integrate the park bench decompression stretch, and "wall-walking" drill, into your walks to accumulate substantial periods of pain-free strides.

A Rounded Upper-Back (Kyphosis): Enhancing Mobility and Correcting the Curve

Several syndromes are associated with a rounding of the upper back – called thoracic hyper-kyphosis. This condition is common among people as they age. Other groups more susceptible to kyphosis include former recreational runners and younger people with habitually poor posture, often linked to texting on the cell phone and sitting too long at the computer or with their tablet in their lap. This postural syndrome causes over-activation of the back muscles, which leads to cramping. It also compromises efficient shoulder motion for overhead work, as well as movements associated with activities like throwing and swimming. Here is a good basic stretch to correct this syndrome, and the associated back and shoulder pain. You will need someone to assist you with this one.

As with all our approaches, stop if you find that this exacerbates your pain. As you gain proficiency, you may perform this on your own using a chair.

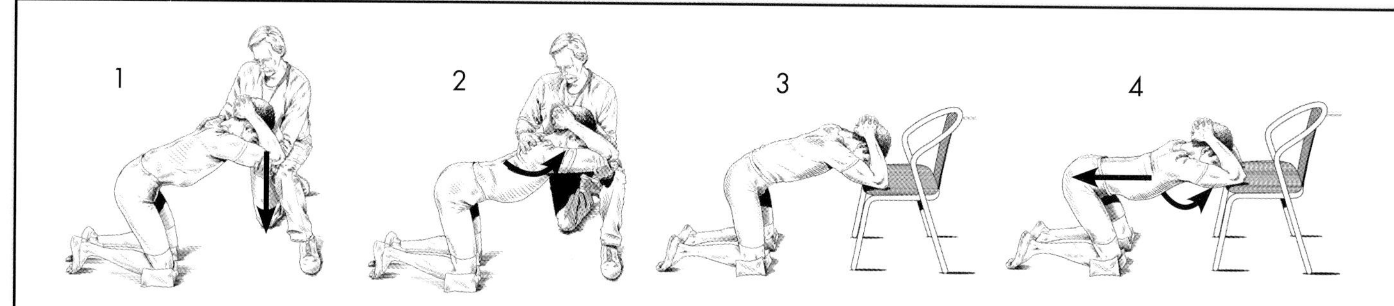

Assisted thoracic extension stretching. You begin by kneeling and positioning the elbows on the clinicians (or assistant's) thigh. The fingers are interlaced and placed behind the head to focus the stretch to the thoracic spine. Rest in this position and ensure that no pain is triggered. Then begin to create a force downwards through the elbows into the assistant of about five pounds (just over two kilos). Hold this exertion for about 10 seconds (1). Then relax. At this time, the assistant "draws" the elbows forwards to allow extension in the thoracic spine (2). This may be repeated up to three times as long as there is a "release" and a noticeable (and pain-free) extension of the thoracic spine.

As you gain proficiency, you may use a chair and a similar technique (3). Instead of an assistant drawing the elbows forwards at the end of the 10 second exertion, pull the buttocks back towards the feet to create the thoracic extension (4).

Repeating this exercise daily will help restore the natural length of your upper spine and aid in alleviating any pain associated with kyphosis.

Mid-Back Pain and the "Chest-Poker" Pattern

Mid-back pain is often associated with a "hinge" in the middle region of the spine. This is to say that these types of patients often use the area of the spine around the base of the ribcage as a focused point for motion and bending. People whose "go-to" posture involves puffing out their ribcage, (in my lab/clinic, we refer to them as "chest-pokers") often complain about mid-back pain. ***This type of pain is merely a symptom of overuse through that section in the spine and can usually be easily alleviated through correcting the habitual postures and movements that force the mid-spine into overdrive.***

How do you know if "chest-poking" is causing your pain? Recall the diagnostic exercise in Section II that involved examining how you "sit up straight". If you find that you move almost exclusively through the ribcage when trying to go from a slouch to an erect position, you are likely a "chest-poker." (Recall chapter 6). If this sounds like you, you may benefit from performing an exercise I've come to refer to as "the Lewit" after the famous Czechoslovakian neurologist Dr. Karel Lewit, whose ideas inspired it. This is an advanced corrective exercise designed to reduce movement in the painful mid-back.

The Lewit: Beginners may wish to work on this exercise with a skilled clinician, but be sure to take this book, as the clinician may not be familiar with this corrective technique. Our goal is to align the spine, avoiding pulling the chest downward which causes stress. Assume a crook-lying posture on the floor, lying on your back with legs off the floor and knees bent at a ninety degree angle. Teeter gently back and forth on the sacrum or tailbone to ease your spine into a neutral position. Place your hands flat, palms down. You may place them under your low back if you are not sure if your spine is in a neutral position. Breathe normally, taking note of your normal inhalation and exhalation lung volumes. This is called "tidal breathing", which has a high tide and a low tide at the end of a normal breath. The exercise begins at low tide. Purse your lips as if blowing through a straw—

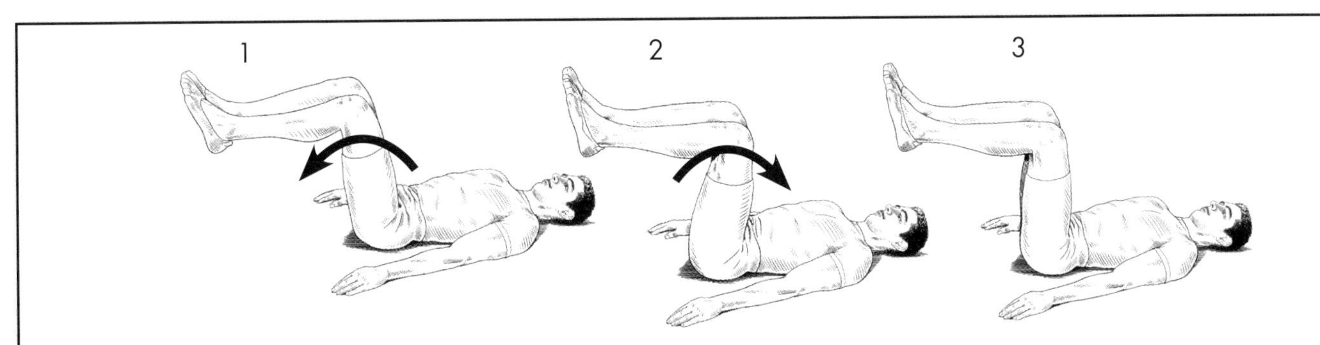

The "Lewit" Setting up the posture: lying on the back, the knees and hips are bent to 90 degrees. (left and middle panel) Mental focus is directed towards "teetering" the pelvis back (1) and forth (2) to obtain the "sweet spot", or pain-free lumbar posture (3). There should be a gap between the lumbar spine and the floor. Some may find benefit from placing the hands, palms down, under the low back.

we want to provide resistance to the breath's airflow. Force air out through pursed lips. Try and get every bit of air out of your lungs. If performed correctly, this exercise activates the abdominal wall and pulls the chest down. In this way, this technique teaches a strategy to combat the "chest poke". Repeat for about three to four cycles. Be forewarned, this can be quite a challenging exercise.

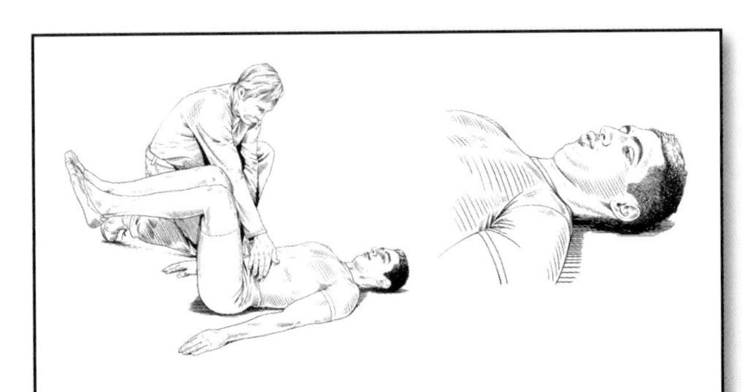

The "Lewit": The exertion begins at the low tide of the breathing cycle. Pursed lips form a tiny hole creating resistance as all air is exhaled from the lungs.

Scoliosis

The most prominent question regarding scoliosis posed by patients and clinicians alike is this: can scoliosis be corrected or assisted with exercise? Further, they want to know if there is a long-term "cure" for resolving scoliosis-related pain. The answer to both questions is, in some cases, yes. There are several theories as to why and how some spines become scoliotic. One is that around the time of pubescent growth (teen years), the spine grows asymmetrically into a lateral curve that may also have some twisting rotation. For some reason, there is often a noticeable difference in the bone density and hardness between the concave and convex sides of the curve. Surgeons will tell you the vertebrae in scoliotic spines feel softer on one side. I have noticed that there is often rib joint asymmetry and even rib unevenness. It is somewhat a case of "the chicken or the egg", in which we are unsure if a rib injury could result in scoliosis, or whether rib issues are byproducts of scoliosis themselves. Whether these anatomical features are cause or effect of the abnormal curves remains unknown.

An important feature of many scoliosis patients is chest and abdominal organ asymmetry. For example, the lung on the concave side of the curve is often smaller with correspondingly smaller volume capacity. While these variances make the treatment strategy more difficult, you may use this feature to your advantage during the corrective exercises.

The fundamental question is, can the curve itself be corrected with exercise? One method of determining the potential for curve reversal involves applying gentle traction (spinal extension) to the back - our preferred technique is to have the patient hang from a bar at arms' length. If, through observation we determine that this position relieves the severity of the curves, the scoliosis has the potential to change with the help of corrective exercise.

Scoliosis Exercises

Scoliosis exercises need to be directed toward the correction of a specific faulty mechanism. If the scoliosis does not seem to be linked to a visible bodily asymmetry, the Schroth method has been helpful for a number of our patients. The approach is based on opening up the concave (or inwardly curved) side with active stretching and breathing. I suggest acquiring a copy of the book, *Three-Dimensional Treatment for Scoliosis* by Christa Lehnert-Schroth.

Scoliosis may have a visible asymmetry such as a short leg, tilting the pelvis down laterally towards the shorter side. A series of heel lifts of increasing height correction is sometimes helpful. Assistance from a skilled clinician is necessary here.

Claudication

People with claudication often mistake their symptoms for stenosis, however claudication is a byproduct of peripheral arterial disease, in other words reduced blood flow of the arteries. Similar to stenosis, claudication makes walking difficult - the longer the walking distance, the greater the difficulty. Walking up stairs usually increases the rate of symptom onset. Here, atherosclerotic plaque buildup narrows the arteries, starving the working leg muscles of oxygen, causing leg pain. A similar approach is used for the claudication patient as for those with stenosis in that walking is trained in tolerable intervals. However, unlike stenosis, I do not know of a preparatory activity prior to walking to increase tolerance. Basically walking is performed until pain becomes moderate. This is one of the few situations where we would allow a patient to work to pain. The patient sits until the symptoms resolve, then resumes walking. Some cardiology associations have set a goal of intervals summing up to 60 minutes three to five times a week. Work with your clinician to see what is best for you.

The Knee or Hip Replacement Patient

These patients have difficulty moving to the floor for exercise. However, spine and core stability is even more important to support the compromised joints. Here we get creative and have the patient standing while performing versions of the "Big 3" stabilization exercises. For example, you are able to perform a version of the bird-dog by bracing a hand/arm on a table or countertop (recall the standing birddog figure in Chapter 11). Front wall planks and rolling into a side wall plank may be a suitable way to begin the progressions. Since the capabilities of each individual will be different, guidance from a skilled clinician may assist here.

The Older Adult

Many of the conditions listed above are more common among older adults (for example stenosis, claudication, kyphosis, etc). The apex of back pain over the life span is typically from age 25 to 55. The good news is that the older adult grows out of having the acute stabs of pain that is characteristic of disc pain. However, the risk is greater for the more arthritic categories of back pain meaning that the recommendations for kyphosis and stenosis are more appropriate. Here are a few features and recommendations specifically for the older adult experiencing back pain.

Osteoporosis is a condition from mineral loss in the vertebra. This leaves them more fragile and likely to fracture during falls, or when lifting heavy weights. Avoiding falls is an important topic and includes preserving the ability to maintain balance and recover from a stumble to arrest the fall. Exercises such as simply standing on one foot, dancing with directional change, and maintaining sufficient hip strength are important for quickly getting the foot planted in front when recovering from a stumble.

Another fact is that many people notice a decline in the ball and socket joints of the shoulders and hips after 50 years of age. Simply, it is more difficult to push loads overhead and to squat deeply. The objective is to perform one or two repetitions of these movements each day just to preserve the ability without flaring up pain symptoms.

Here is a suggestion for a program that has been practiced by many wise older adults who have aged successfully:

1. Incorporate the "joint sparing" movement tools (squat, lunge, and stop-twist) into daily activity.
2. Get up early each morning and get your chores done.
3. Walk 2 times per day, each day.
4. Do some strength training 2 days per week.
5. Do something different 2 days per week (bike, swim etc).
6. Work on mobility in areas that need this 3 days per week.
7. Encourage good sleep with less alcohol consumption.

The Overweight Patient

If you fall into this category, you're probably sick of doctors advising you to slim down. Unfortunately, reality television programs about weight-loss are unrepresentative of what is usually possible, even in a successful program. ***The reality for your back, is that being at a healthy body weight will aid tremendously in eliminating or reducing pain.*** Those of you with weight issues may have been conditioned to fail through previous unsuccessful weight-loss attempts. To succeed here you will need a strong support system to help you to comply with the clinical exercise prescription. That being said, your success will depend first and foremost on your ability to curb over-eating and make better food choices.

Once body weight is reduced, then simple exercise progressions are commenced with good form (corrected walking, and simple starting levels of the spine sparing drills). Although a currently overweight patient can begin with the programs outlined in this book, they will experience greater success with a coupled focus on weight reduction.

Interestingly, I have not found very heavy people with spine instability as their girth is naturally stabilizing. Thus, with them, we focus more on performing work to enhance endurance and strength in the patterns of movement noted earlier. Exercises for stabilization such as the "Big 3", one-legged exercise and stretching are de-emphasized.

Chapter 15

Solutions that Solve Back Pain: Case Studies and Sample Programs

Solutions that Solve Back Pain

Case Studies and Sample Programs

Remember that although the majority of you reading this book will benefit from following the core exercise program outlined in Section III, this is not a "one-size-fits-all" recovery plan. It must be modified and adjusted to fit each individual's limitations while avoiding their personal pain triggers. Rarely does one fit perfectly into a back pain category. In fact, some of you possess traits from several categories. You are encouraged to read a few of the case studies below to glean some hints that may help you to better understand your own unique symptoms as well as gain further suggestions for reducing your pain. Doing this should help to "fine tune" the links between what you discovered about your back pain in the assessment section and applying your best solution given your unique circumstances.

The "typical recovery" experience goes like this:

- Make a conscious effort to eliminate the pain triggers.

- The "Big 3" exercises are then adapted into the daily schedule and become increasingly easier. Little by little, tasks that once caused pain become pain-free.

- More exercises are added as the pain-free repertoire expands. Somewhere around this stage in recovery, an individual can get a little overzealous and tries to add in a new activity only to find that pain has returned the next day. Although it's important to continue to expand your abilities, it is possible to do too much too soon. It is important to look at these moments as lessons.

- You now have a better sense of your current limits at this stage in your improvement.

- If the progress momentum has been lost, you should regress back to a lesser challenge, one that worked before. You will find that you regain the pain-free ability faster this time and that you don't have to start at "square one".

- You will likely repeat this scenario a few times, experiencing the occasional set-back, until you ultimately become pain-free.

Each case study will be presented in three parts:

1. His/her/their story
2. What not to do
3. What to do

Matt has a painful stiff back most mornings

His story

Matt wakes up just about every morning with the type of back stiffness that makes putting on his socks for work a nightmare. What's the typical advice someone like Matt receives? To stretch. He's told to pull the knees to the chest, hold them there and work the stiffness out. If this is what you do, STOP THIS! STOP THIS NOW! You, like Matt, may have experienced temporary relief via the back muscle stretch reflex for about 15 minutes, but this type of stretching will ensure that you will have stiffness tomorrow and every day after that.

What not to do

Matt should not stretch. And, like Matt, do not sleep on a futon or a soft floppy mattress that allows the torso to sink curving the spine. Do not sleep with a pillow under the knees.

What to do

Matt often travels for work. He has found that after sleeping in some of these beds that he miraculously wakes in the morning with no back pain. Has this happened to you? If so, both you and Matt should check your mattress.

The shape of your spine will help you choose the best mattress. Typically those of you who have more lumbar lordosis (hollow curve), protruding buttocks, or more curves, will have more mattress-related pain. For you, lying on the back is problematic. Your body shape forces your spine to be suspended and unsupported like the middle part of a bridge. This, in turn, pushes the lumbar spine into flexion as it flattens to the mattress, causing pain and stiffness. For individuals with this type of body,

I would recommend NOT sleeping on a futon. A mattress that allows the buttocks to sink in helps. Choosing a firm mattress with a quality foam topper should provide the ideal combination of support and cushion. I have also created a sleeping back support with my colleagues. "The McGill Sleeper" can be seen at www.backfitpro.com. The support is adjusted with a hand pump to reduce stress and pain for a variety of mattresses and spine shapes.

Placing a pillow under the knees can actually be problematic as it adds to the flattening of the lumbar spine into the mattress. That being said, side sleepers may appreciate placing a pillow between their knees to alleviate strain on the hips. "Peanut shaped" pillows are available for this purpose.

After rising from bed, avoid spine flexion as much as possible. The best way to achieve this is to use a pair of slip-on shoes and go for a walk before sitting down for morning coffee. Do a few cat-camel cycles to move the back, avoiding pushing to the end range of motion. Perform the "Big 3" exercises later in the morning. Walk several more times during the day.

Build the number of reps/sets slowly. If pain remains an issue, scale back your routine. Don't put yourself in overdrive in an effort to progress at a quicker rate. Consider exercising in shorter intervals, performing a smaller portion of the exercise, splitting up your sets and completing them in another session later in the day. Always stay within your pain tolerance.

Pamela's pain ramps up throughout the day

Her story

Pamela is a business boomer. She's self-employed, works from home and juggles a hectic schedule that includes her kids, volunteering and training for her first half marathon. Pam wakes up every morning with very little pain and next to no back issues. In fact, the morning is the best part of her day. As her busy day wears on however, her back pain increases. This indicates that cumulative loading on Pam's spine is exceeding her pain-free tolerance. Does this sound familiar?

What not to do

Do not keep going as you are. The key in Pam's and perhaps your situation is to remove the offending motions, postures and loads that accumulate and result in pain and more pain. Also you and Pam must reduce the duration of each offending task by adding more spine unloading breaks.

What to do

First, ensure that your symptoms have begun to wind down following a course of good spine hygiene. This also means incorporating spine conserving movements and more frequent rest breaks. You and Pam should experience a reduction of symptoms typically after just a few days. At this point, begin the basic spine rehab program outlined earlier. This will produce a higher capacity for pain-free living.

Alisha is the typical type "A" personality (the go-getter and keen exerciser)

Her story

When someone like Alisha, a typical type A personality, is given a program with 10 repetitions of an exercise, she will always do more, maybe 20 repetitions. She believes more is always better. She thinks that she can crush the pain with more work. In fact, sadly it is exactly this approach that keeps Alisha in pain. Sound like anyone else you know?

What not to do

Continue to believe that the pain will be "exercised" away and that more is better.

What to do

With this classic type "A" personality, I like to play this game: I ask Alisha to pretend that today she actually had surgery to cure her back – now tomorrow she will start her recovery. And by recovery, I mean rest. This ensures a program that removes all loading to give the overstressed and painful components time off. As I have already stated, surgery often works initially because it forces the patient to simply rest. The reduction in symptoms clearly demonstrates the efficiency of this approach.

Typically, patients like Alisha fear they will lose their fitness so they will continue to overexert their backs. These are the people who work out every day for an hour or more. You know the type. So, if you're an Alisha and love to win, try playing the "virtual surgery" game, because chances are it will deliver a win!

Brad is the type "B" personality (he does not like to exercise)

His story

Brad is 55, has had the same accounting job for 15 years where he sits at his desk all day, then drives home, has dinner and then spends most evenings on the sofa with his computer on his lap. Brad and his type "B" personality is the polar opposite to Alisha and her type "A" behaviours. It is not unusual for "B" types like Brad to have multiple conditions of diabetes, obesity and/or muscle weakness. They are activity adverse and enjoy the comforts of eating and reclining while watching TV. When Brad is given a movement program with 10 repetitions, you can put money on it that he'll stop at three. Brad and "B" types everywhere need motivation to push on and enjoy a pain-free life. Brad finds excuse after excuse and will often use more energy complaining about his condition than he would need to actually start improving it.

What not to do

If you're a Brad, stop getting in your own way. Stop complaining about pain if you're not prepared to act. Stop making excuses. Stop spending so much time sitting at work when you could walk around the office or take a walk on your lunch break. Stop spending so much time on the sofa when you could take the dog for a walk. Plan other activities into tolerable intervals.

What to do

This may sound harsh, but the stark reality is Brad "deserves" his pain – he has brought it upon himself. When it comes to dealing with his pain, he has a choice – he can avoid the exercises and live a painful, sedentary, miserable life 24 hours a day or he can take action and dedicate himself to a daily training session of at least an hour to help improve the other 23 hours he has every day.

I present the "Brads" I see with a choice. If they choose to assist themselves, I help them 100%. If they don't, I suggest that I am unable to help them – but I leave them with the offer that if they change their minds I will be available. Some continue to seek out a guru who will offer them an easy "cure" – almost always remaining pained, fragile, and unable to enjoy pain-free activity.

Dave – the more he drives, the more pain he experiences

His story

Dave is a truck driver by trade and he has been noticing lately that his back and leg pains increase in direct proportion with the amount of driving he does. Dave's pain may be a combination of ischemia (clogged blood supply) and back trouble. When trying to differentiate between the two, keep this in mind: ischemic pain resolves once out of the vehicle, but back pain lingers.

What not to do

For truckers or taxi drivers or anyone who drives a great deal, do not keep your wallet and other objects in your back pockets. Do not wear tight and constrictive clothing. Do not wear heels, as these will compound your back grief when trying to walk. And, most importantly, Dave, do not continue driving for long periods without periodic rest and stretch breaks.

What to do

Use the basic back fitness plan outlined in this book. Adjusting the seat to support a neutral posture often helps. Increase the angle between the seat pan and the seat back by reclining slightly. This helps reduce the flexion pressure on the spine and relaxes the hip tissues. Dave may want to use a lumbar support/cushion to reduce back stress (a rolled up towel will work although an adjustable "Lumbair" (www.backfitpro.com) is best). Dave should also take breaks from driving; get out of the driver's seat and practice the standing McGill stretch (see chapter 8). Then he should go for a brisk walk before getting back in the driver's seat.

Penny experiences the majority of her pain through her buttocks and in her posterior thigh. She's the misdiagnosed "Piriformis syndrome" patient.

Her story

Penny can specifically trace the path of her pain from her hip joint, through the leg-pelvis crease, deep through the posterior of the buttocks down the bone in the back of her thigh and all the way down to her toes. This is sometimes misdiagnosed as "piriformis syndrome," which is actually a very rare condition. The pain is almost always caused by lumbar nerve root irritation. Recall our section on sciatica. If the pain is felt in the big toe, then the L5 root is the problematic level. Likewise, pain in the other toes points to the L4 lumbar level. Penny should check for gluteal muscle weakness (see the self-assessment chapter). Penny also experiences tightness in her hamstrings. She's tried stretching them over a period of time and has failed to relax the muscle tension.

What not to do

Do not continue stretching the hip and the hamstrings (and sciatic nerve) as nerve pain cannot be stretched away—by doing this you are actually increasing sensitivity!

What to do

Move in a spine-sparing way that will unload the pressure on the lumbar joints. This means practicing good spine hygiene throughout the day. As the pain triggers are removed, pain sensitivity winds down. If the nerve-pinch is related to the disc, then sitting with a lumbar support usually helps. Take frequent breaks (use the McGill standing stretch from Chapter 8 to break up periods of prolonged sitting). Develop your walking program based on the tolerable interval system. Adjusting head and neck posture is also an important factor in reducing the pinch. If you have found that the lying-on-the-tummy-supporting-the-chin-with-fists posture helps, continue to incorporate this posture into your day. It is particularly effective if performed right before a walk. Nerve flossing may also help (see chapter 14).

Pete finds that exercise stimulates pain into his buttocks and the front of his thigh

His story

Pete is similar to Penny, only Pete's pain is experienced down the front of the thigh. Pete loves playing soccer, but his pain is increased with kicking a ball or with activities that load the spine (like stacking wood at the cottage). If the pain is more medial (down the inside of the thigh), Pete should have his hips assessed as they are the possible culprits. Otherwise, anterior thigh pain is likely due to lumbar joint pathology at the L3 level or higher (this usually suggests femoral nerve root impingement and pain).

What not to do

Pete needs to stop irritating the hips and spine with poor quality movement and too much activity that loads the spine. Unfortunately, this means less soccer for Pete, at least temporarily. He will slowly rebuild his pain tolerance for this type of exercise through corrective movement.

What to do

For patients like Pete, lying on the stomach and proceeding to flex the knees often worsens the pain. If you find this to be true to your case, follow the general plan for the posterior thigh pain patient in the previous example. If the hip is the primary pain generator, you will need to find the optimal dose of activity, not too much or too little, that minimizes pain. Also, try the hip therapeutic exercise program already introduced in this book.

Cameron and his computer work (he who sits at work)

His story

Cameron is a 35-year-old office worker who sits at a computer for eight to ten hours a day. Accustomed to sitting slouched, when Cameron sits upright he has no pain. Through self-observation, Cameron can pinpoint the discs in his back that cause his problems. His painful spine segments are easily identified. The "McKenzie posture" (quiet lying on the stomach), takes pain away. His pain is in his low back, over the sacroiliac joints (the dimples on either side of the spine base). He also occasionally experiences bursts of pain in the back of his thighs. When not sitting for hours on end at work, he likes to lie around watching TV on a couch or sit in his Lazy-Boy playing video games. When asked to squat, Cameron naturally bends his knees and his spine. This man has tight hip flexors, poor core endurance and an inability to engage his gluteal muscles.

What not to do

Cameron needs to stop sitting for prolonged periods both at home and at work. He needs to stop merely *hoping* that passive therapies are the answer. He will break the cycle of pain when he builds corrective exercise into his schedule and chooses not to be governed by a sedentary lifestyle.

What to do

Cameron needs to get out of the chair regularly and use the McGill Stretch (previous section). When at the office, he should sit with a Lumbair support and use his lunch breaks to go for a brisk walk. Practice the "Big 3" exercises and employ walking lunges (see chapter 12) to reduce the tension in the hip flexors and alleviate this pain. In addition, Cameron must improve his health with more, and better, chosen activities. End of story.

Octavio the opera singer – when back pain jeopardizes your career

His story

Octavio, who has a flexion intolerant lumbar disc, needed more torso stiffness and stability to control his pain. He was successful in creating sufficient stiffness for pain control through strength training but the stiffness radiated to his shoulders and neck, inhibiting his breathing and vocal power. In fact, the breath-holding patterns he had developed while strength training had actually caused his diaphragm to open his esophageal sphincter (the muscle controlling the opening to the stomach). This led to nighttime acid reflux that further compromised his voice.

What not to do

Octavio needs to stop his weight training and his exaggerated breathing. He also needs to stop over-stiffening his abdominal muscles. In an effort to properly brace his core, he has gone too far.

What to do

Over-bracing of the abdominal and torso muscles can cause several disorders. Simultaneous over-activation of the diaphragm can affect stomach function together with breathing efficiency. Stiffening and bracing must be tuned to the individual situation – there is no "right way" that works for everyone. Octavio needs to learn to stiffen the lower torso while relaxing the upper torso. This means adjusting the abdominal brace while relaxing the chest with each breath. These patterns are repeated to ingrain this pattern for training and daily activity. The side plank while breathing deeply can assist Octavio with this.

Loretta is oblivious to her body postures and movements

Her story

Loretta is like so many of the people I observe. Although she's 33, she's never really tried to know her own body and never been aware of her lazy posture or her less than efficient body movements. It still amazes me to this day the variance in humans regarding the trait of body awareness. I don't know if this is a "modern" condition as people have become less reliant on their movement efficiency to survive. I suspect that not too many centuries ago they would have been eliminated from the gene pool by the physical dangers of the times or from the inability to forage for food. With these individuals, when I begin coaching the abdominal brace to stiffen the torso and say, "stiffen your abdominals as if you were to be punched in the stomach." They respond, "How do I do that?" I must have gone to a different kind of school!

What not to do

Loretta and others like her need to stop ignoring their own anatomy. As with any high performance machine, there is a right and a wrong way to treat it for peak performance. Loretta needs to cease her sloppy posture and mindless movements.

What to do

For people like Loretta, I teach a foundation for movement starting with having her grasp my hand and squeeze. No movement occurs, only an increase in force and stiffness. Progressively we work through the body regions creating exertional force against immobile objects. This establishes "proximal stiffness," which enables efficient movement and power development at the shoulders and hips. We then practice torso stiffening and tuning of the "abdominal brace". We begin simple movements such as the "hip hinge" and the movement patterns shown in the previous sections. We may utilize some of the progressive movement teaching techniques shown earlier. As Loretta becomes aware of her movement strategies, she will become better able to solve painful movements with this mindful approach.

Samina and Sadie are both stenosis patients

Their story

Both Samina and Sadie's back pains have driven them to adopt a hunched position. They find walking and exercise in general to be painful and their pains often radiate down their legs. Although both women have stenosis, the direct cause of their pains vary. Remember that the diagnosis of stenosis indicates a narrowing of the nerve canals that impinge the nerve itself. The source of the compression could be, such as in Sadie's case, a bulging disc. In Samina's situation it could be an arthritic bone, or a number of other ailments including a hypertrophied facet capsule or ligament, or an anatomical anomaly. Because there are different causes of stenosis, each example will be addressed with a prevention and rehabilitation plan individually.

What not to do AND what to do

Samina's Situation - Stenosis with arthritis

Samina, at 76 is a perfect example. Her type of stenosis usually occurs in an older individual where arthritic bone has grown into the spaces where nerve roots travel, or perhaps the disc has flattened due to previous vertebral or disc injury. Nonetheless, Samina's ability to walk is usually limited to short distances. Yet walking is essential to general and spine health. Poor movement patterns such as bending the spine instead of hip hinging throughout the day have further sensitized her back, compounding the pain sensitivity. Obviously spine hygiene is appropriate here as with all back conditions. Samina should practice patterns of corrected walking to reduce any pain, and try different arm swing patterns (see chapter 8). In general, she should walk faster and with purpose, but stop short of producing symptoms. After her walk, she should assume a healthy relaxed position such as the "wall-walk" outlined earlier. If this reduces the symptoms, then walk in a park where benches are available for this drill. Walk for a few minutes at a time and practice this drill on the bench. Keep repeating this exercise to successfully achieve a pain-free walking session. Soon, walking will, in many cases, become tolerable again.

Sadie's case - Stenosis with a disc bulge

Sadie, age 48, has played a more direct role in causing her stenosis. Recall that focal disc bulges result from specific movements. First, Sadie needs to remove the offending movement patterns that caused the bulge and it will most likely resorb and return to a healthy disc – refer back to the assessment chapter. These "disc corrections" may also be performed at strategic times. For example, if Sadie knows that when she lies in bed she experiences radiating symptoms from a disc bulge, she should try lying on her tummy for a few minutes first. Note that this will not work with the arthritic spine. Sadie needs to find bulge reducing postures, consider nerve flossing, and adopt the approaches described in chapter 14.

Stenosis with a flattened disc

Generally, minimizing spine motion works best to relieve this type of pain. Focus all of your movements around the hip joints instead, and employ the movement tools introduced in chapters 7 and 8.

The bizarre pained patient

There are the "bizarre" patients who are dismissed as being "nuts". Here are a few stories that you may relate to if you have been through the medical system and failed to get better, and worse, if you were made to feel as though your "failure" was your fault. I will group them together and forgo the format of the previous examples.

I have seen too many patients discarded in the heap and labeled as "bizarre" or "non-compliant", or they are dismissed with the all too familiar, "your pain is in your head."

This is terribly unfortunate, and usually results from a lack of medical expertise and poor diagnostic skill. While spine pain is simple to manage in many people, it can be very complex in others. For example, I had one patient referred to me with back pain, but she complained of related "crotch pain" (her words). She had great difficulty walking, particularly up stairs. Our examination revealed that her traumatic injury during a car accident had erased the movement engrams (or "muscle memory") that reside in the spinal cord at the level of the damage. This was not visible on any of her x-rays and she was dismissed as a nut. She had to "think" about walking again, re-teaching herself the patterns and repeating them with mindful concentration so they became once again ingrained, default patterns. Her back pain slowly resolved with the resumption of normal movements. The arrogant medics who had labeled her a "nut" dismissed our successful treatments as "luck."

I have had four patients over my career with "muscle resonance". Here, the abdominal muscles quiver and vibrate with certain exertions, such as bending or rising from a chair. They vibrate at a frequency known as neural resonance (about 8 to 10 cycles per second). Every one of these patients had trauma to the T9, or T10 vertebral level – the level that provides nerve innervation to the abdominal muscles, particularly the Rectus Abdominis muscle. These were difficult cases, and half of them responded to the general approaches outlined in this book – the other two failed to improve. That's 50% saved of patients who were written off by the medical community.

Some patients who have baffled the traditional medics display "paradoxical signs," where one symptom suggests a specific disorder while the next symptom suggests the opposite. For example, lying on your back and raising a leg causes back and thigh pain, which suggests an irritated nerve root, but raising the head with forward neck bend reduces pain (note: this usually increases pain), suggesting no neural tension. In this case, a bulged disc had formed an "underhook" on the nerve root so that leg movement pulled the nerve into the disc bulge while neck movement pulled the nerve off the disc bulge. A traditional assessment did not assist here. Only an assessment in which tests were based on clinical logic rather than typical "form tests" led to the uncovering of this mechanism. Spine hygiene practices cured this patient. As crazy as it sounds, you will probably be better at finding the solution yourself by following this guide.

Cases of "pain allodynia" illustrate the injustice resulting from medical examinations by non-experts. Allodynia is a name for extreme sensitivity to pain. One sufferer I encountered could not bear the weight of a summer bed sheet resting on his toes. One medic suggested foot amputation, while another "determined" that the pain was in his head. During our examination, we found a lumbar nerve trap from a bulging disc which was released with a flossing routine and spine hygiene program. We found that his bulge grew when in prolonged spine flexion postures and shrank in extension postures. Once he figured this out he was able to cure himself. He is quite fine today, has both of his feet, and is a pillar of his community—far from being a nutcase.

There are also the fibromyalgic cases who are often dismissed by back doctors. Pains are reported as "swirly" and "scratchy" in nature, often over the hip and shoulder regions. Headache and back pain are often a part of the equation. I am convinced that the pain is real and that it is related to the brain being "rewired" to perceive the pain differently. Both pain perception and body movements are encoded patterns in the brain. Quite often these patients have been traumatized in violent events such as a car crash or during a very intense emotional incident. This can cause the brain to immediately rewire a pattern that changes how pain is generated and perceived. The approach that has produced the best results for us over the years has been to teach the patient pain-free movement. This is based on the "gate theory" of pain. Finding simple movements that do not cause pain, floods the proprioceptive system with joint and muscle sensor signals, leaving little room for pain signals to get through the neural "gates". These pain-free movements are repeated to encode the pattern in the brain. Slowly the patient's repertoire of pain-free movement increases until they are able to move well, and for longer periods. They successfully replaced the pain inducing patterns wired into their brains with pain-free patterns.

All of the case studies above, together with hundreds more, had consults with "spine experts". All these patients had failed to find the true cause, and relief. They were made to feel that either their painful predicament was their own fault or was due to their mental or emotional weakness. You see they had not seen a true expert. Having come this far in this book, you are the back mechanic, you are an expert in perceiving your pains, understanding their cause, and finding effective strategies to relieve them.

You will find many more "case studies" of athletic examples in my book *"Ultimate Back Fitness and Performance."*

Chapter 16

Q and A Time With the Back Mechanic: Sex, Selecting a Mattress and Other Things You Were Afraid to Ask

Q and A Time With the Back Mechanic

Sex, Selecting a Mattress and Other Things You Were Afraid to Ask

Some days I awake to find a couple of hundred email messages from doctors, patients and athletes seeking advice. I have compiled some of the most interesting, or commonly asked questions here in this last chapter. Some of these points may be repetitive, some new, some providing a slightly different perspective, but they are all shared here in the interest of providing a more complete answer. My answers also focus only on the spine-related elements rather than other factors presented in the broader questions.

By now you are savvy to the idea that no one else will "fix" your back for you – you must be an active participant in the healing process. Putting together the details for your specific case will give you the tools to live the best life possible, one free from back pain. The reality is that some back injuries will take years for the damaged tissue to heal but after reading this book, you are now skilled in managing damage to sub-clinical levels. You are enjoying life again!

Will ergonomic design in my workplace help my back?

Ergonomics is the science of designing the job to fit the worker. Modifications such as optimizing the layout of an assembly job by eliminating the need to pick up objects from the floor can really help spare the backs of the workers. This is of particular importance for the older worker whose hips are a bit stiffer. But how can a forestry job, or construction trade, or work on a fishing vessel be ergonomically designed? Put simply, they can't. All the worker can do is choose how they will move and load their bodies to spare the muscles and joints. I have developed the concept of "job coaching". Job coaching has two components: optimizing the design of the work with ergonomic principles together with coaching the worker regarding movements to avoid overuse injury. In summary, the influence of ergonomic job design to cure a painful back varies depending upon the job. Yes, it can help, but success requires the dual approach of job design and coaching the worker to move in spine friendly ways.

You talk about spine hygiene all day long – what do you mean?

Spine hygiene means sparing your back in all activities during the day. This accomplishes two things: the individual has longer periods without pain, and the back has more capacity to tolerate training with appropriate exercise to become more resilient. Look at every task and do not dismiss the importance of this concept. How do you tie your shoes – flexing the spine? Many people sit down and reach for their foot using up a bend cycle that could be saved for a therapeutic activity. Instead, put the foot up on the chair or bench and lunge towards the foot with the torso upright, keeping the spine in a neutral position, moving the hips towards the foot to reduce the reach distance (recall figure in chapter 8). Sitting, bending, walking, driving, etc. are all opportunities to practice good spine hygiene. Remember that achieving and maintaining back health is a full-time activity, a way of life, where awareness of your own movements is of the upmost importance.

Do you have tips for travelling?

Travelling has the potential to provide several roadblocks on the journey to recovery, including poorly designed airplane seats, strange beds, disruption from a regular routine and either a potential increase or decrease in the amount of daily walking. I do not know why airline seats are designed with a hollow in the lumbar region – the precise opposite of having a lumbar support. A few years ago we did a study on the spine stresses that develop from sitting in airplane seats and we could not get an answer as to why they almost seemed designed to damage backs. The solution here is to carry on a lumbar pad or pillow. A visit to www.backfitpro.com will show you an inflatable lumbar pad measured to reduce airline seat stress. Also, it is wise to stand and walk the aisles periodically, purposefully exaggerating the lumbar lordosis or hollow curve in the back. When you arrive at your destination, it is a good idea to walk around before picking up your luggage; do not resume sitting while you wait. Stroll and focus on returning the normal hollow in your back. This will better prepare you to lift your suitcase without injury and pain.

Different beds can be a blessing or a curse. Sleeping in an unfamiliar bed allows some people to experiment and see if the change in firmness causes them to be more or less stiff in the morning. Be cognizant of the hardness of the mattress itself together with the amount of "pillow top" or cushioning on the top. If you find the bed has reduced your pain, note the make and model, maybe it's time to replace your mattress at home.

A final thought should be given about staying on routine with the "Big 3" exercises. The beauty is that they can be performed anywhere. Push-ups can be performed in a hotel room along with your stabilization routine. Short walks are also easily accommodated. Certainly be conscious of the time spent sitting in meetings. Use your Lumbair and stand frequently. Encourage your meeting mates to do the same – they will enjoy the relief as well.

How do I choose a bed mattress and pillow?

Now that we have introduced the issue of beds, your job is to find the best one for you. If you wake and rise and are stiff most mornings, then have a look at your mattress as a contributing factor to your pain. Scientific studies provide some guidance here. As with many back issues, they are specific to the individual. For example, research shows that some cultures sleep on a futon and find it comfortable. Generally they have a flatter back with less lordosis (a characteristic of some Asian spines). Other cultures find futons uncomfortable, and, as expected, have more lordosis as a population (some European and African spines). More research has divided body types into angular and bonier groups versus rounder groups that carry more body weight. Bodies with more curves will do better with a firm foundation but a cushioned top that allows the curvy hips and shoulders to sink in. A thicker pillow top is helpful here. A heavier person with less defined curves would do better in a firmer bed altogether.

Selecting a pillow depends on the type of dominant sleeping position. A stomach sleeper may wish to not use a pillow. A back sleeper may want only minimal support under the neck. For those who alternate between back and side, they will be better supported with a specialty pillow that has little material in the middle (for back sleeping) and bolstered wings that support the head when the individual rolls over for side sleeping. Finally, some back sleepers will benefit from the low back support "McGill sleeper" noted previously (available on www.backfitpro.com).

What is the best sleeping posture?

There is no definitive answer. However the guiding principle remains – avoid what hurts you. Some disc patients with spine flexion intolerance do well as stomach sleepers. This would be impossible for many older arthritic spines. Those who prefer to lie on their backs and are provoked with spine flexion can find relief by placing a small pad in the lumbar area to prevent it from flattening and flexing into the mattress. Some others believe that side sleeping in a fetal position is more comfortable, and yet when they undergo provocative testing they find spine flexion to actually be one of their triggers! Armed with this information, they try to have some hip flexion but a neutral lumbar spine in order to modify their favorite sleeping position so that their pain trigger is avoided. Interestingly, for back sleepers with hip pain, having a pillow under the knees is helpful, while many with back pain find this method only aggravates their symptoms.

What about back belts?

No doubt many of you have seen athletes on TV wearing back belts, or workers using them when lifting, and have wondered if they are for you. People generally use these because they want to alleviate their back pain, or increase their weight training capacity. These "belts" were more common years ago but waned in popularity as the science developed. Our lab was responsible for several of the initial investigations that really questioned many of the claims supporting belt wearing. Having stated this, there are circumstances where temporary belt wearing may help.

There have been several claims made to justify back belts. They:

- remind people to lift properly.
- support shear loading on the spine.
- reduce compressive loading (minimally) of the lumbar spine.
- act as a splint on the torso, reducing the range of motion and thereby decreasing the risk of injury.
- provide warmth to the lumbar region.
- enhance awareness via pressure to increase the perception of stability.
- reduce muscular fatigue.
- provide stiffening to the torso to enhance performance.

Some of these claims proved to be valid and others did not stand true when tested in the lab. Through our testing, we were able to draw several conclusions about the effectiveness of these devices. The majority of the scientific evidence regarding the use of a belt comes from occupational settings. A review of the effects of wearing a belt in occupational settings suggests that:

- Those who do not have a previous back injury appear to have no additional protective benefit from wearing a belt.
- Those who are injured while wearing a belt seem to risk a more severe injury.
- Belts appear to give people the perception they can lift more and in many cases may in fact enable them to lift more – belts do assist in supplying lifting forces.
- Belts appear to increase intra-abdominal pressure and blood pressure. This is both good and bad.
- Belts appear to change the lifting styles of some people - either decreasing or increasing the loads on the spine, depending on the individual.
- When a habitual belt-wearer suddenly discontinues its use, there is a period of higher risk of injury. This suggests that some physiological/neurological changes occur during long-term belt wearing.

When deciding whether or not to use a belt, consider the following: if you are an athlete wishing to lift maximum weight, then wear a belt. It will help you lift a few more pounds (or kilos) through elastic recoil effects and by adding stiffness to the spine. If you merely want to enhance your back health and are not attempting maximum lifts, then it is better not to wear one.

Having stated this, there are some patients who experience pain when walking and lifting that is reduced with compression of the pelvic ring. These individuals sometimes benefit from wearing a belt lower around the pelvis not around the waist. This is a temporary measure until the rehabilitation exercises ("Big 3" for example) strengthen and stiffen the pelvic ring.

For others, the belt temporarily assists with pain-free walking and bending. Here is the issue—belts will never cure back pain. I was asked to write the policy on belt wearing for several governments and company health departments in the early '90's. The essence of my recommendations were clear: belt wearing as a company-wide policy for those performing demanding work is not justifiable. However, if an individual gets temporary benefit from a belt, the essential elements of the policy were as follows:

1. They get an ergonomic assessment of their job to optimize layout to spare their joints.
2. They receive a mandatory education program regarding spine sparing principles and, what to do if they think they have re-injured themselves.
3. They have a health exam to ensure there is no pre-existing cardiovascular compromise since belt wearing will adjust blood pressure and intra-abdominal pressure.
4. They undergo a back assessment that determines their movement flaws and pain mechanism, which is then addressed appropriately.
5. They commit to a therapeutic exercise program to develop the natural anatomic belt that each of us has, and they must continue the program long after they are weaned from the belt given that this is a period of higher injury risk.

So should I really stop stretching? I enjoy it!

For many, stretching early in a pain reduction program usually causes more back trouble than it cures – particularly those that involve bending through the spine. Recall that static stretching (that is reaching and holding a stretch), when tested, has not been shown to reduce injury as had been its previous claim. In fact, those with greater spine mobility, and flexibility in particular, are actually a higher risk category for future back pain. I will again return to the idea that while many experience a temporary relief after stretching, this is due to a stimulation of the stretch reflex and is only a fleeting mask of the damage you are causing underneath. This is not to say that no type of stretch is ever beneficial in any way, but I would simply warn you to be very judicious when deciding whether or not to stretch. You must have a specific reason. For example, if increased hip mobility is the goal, decide on the best way to achieve this. Perhaps a selection of more dynamic exercise would be the more appropriate course of action. By this I mean exercise that moves the joint continuously such as the walking lunge, as opposed to a static stretch that is pushed to an end range and held still. That being said, there are some who will benefit from thoracic extension mobility stretches such as the partnered exercise where you rest your elbows on another's thigh.

This stretch is particularly helpful for those needing corrections to their standing posture, or who are hunched over with age. In summary, stretching must be justified and have a clear intent. For example, practicing yoga for mobility will compromise the stiffness needed to lift heavy weights. It is not possible to be a yoga master and be a champion powerlifter. Further, stretching technique matters and must be well executed to ensure that it is therapeutic and not actually worsening your condition. In summary, leave stretching for later in the program progression.

What about gym balls, bands, weights and machines?

There are all kinds of exercise toys and gadgets. Except for some of the advanced exercises, the program described here uses none of them. I have access to any back rehab device that I want, but I choose not to use any of them, simply because I don't feel they are a necessary component in a patient's recovery. Generally, when performing exercises to eliminate pain we avoid gadgets. It is much better to train the body to move well and become fitter using its own weight. Once pain is gone and the training transitions to enhance function and athleticism, then fitness "accessories" can be reintroduced. Again, the use of these gadgets for specific progressions of training is described in my book, *"Ultimate Back Fitness and Performance"*.

Do I really need to exercise every day?

Yes! Absolutely! Without question! Your body thrives on daily work and needs this for its overall health. The idea of "working out" three times per week was based on a body-building philosophy regarding the hypertrophying (or "bulking") of muscle. This body-building practice had nothing to do with the health of your musculoskeletal system. The notion of reaching a training heart rate 3-4 times per week is also a myth. This one happens to be perpetuated by the aerobics community and is not applicable to the average person trying to reduce back pain. Also, keep in mind that our daily training sessions outlined in this book for back patients should not resemble anything close to a "workout" being performed by someone in the gym trying to get "skinny" or obtain muscular bulk. Instead, our daily exercise routines, particularly for those just beginning their recovery, are focused on taking incremental steps towards building a solid base of pain-free living. Furthermore, our most recent work has shown that performing the "Big 3" exercises every day creates a lasting stiffness in the spine joints that inhibit the pain-causing micro-movements. Perform the routine that you have gleaned from this book every day – even twice per day! Quoting my friend Pavel Tsatsouline, "a good workout leaves you with more than it takes away".

I have painful knees. What can I do?

Painful knees prevent people from kneeling on the floor to perform exercises like the bird-dog. You could try kneepads. Those used in indoor volleyball offer great padding and may be enough to allow you to perform these exercises. Alternate forms of the exercises can really help here. For the bird-dog, try performing it in a standing position supporting yourself on a high-level table (recall chapter 9). Remember that side-bridges can also be modified to be performed standing (see chapter 9). Work with what you have. A clever clinician will assess your capabilities and restrictions and figure out a plan to modify your program while directly addressing the original cause of your knee pain.

What should I do if I reinjure myself?

The fact is that many back injuries do not recover like others. Consider a broken leg. The bones mend themselves, forming a strong fusion and do not present a weak spot in the future. Back disorders, however, can rarely be healed short-term and then forgotten about. Instead, they must be managed. The truth is that most patients will experience a minor relapse at some point in their recovery and will feel some of their symptoms returning. If you have a history of disc pain, for example and have just poorly executed a lift, you may begin to feel an acute attack coming on. Identify these early signs of a relapse and combat them by lying on the tummy with one fist under the chin. We have shown this posture can reverse the impending disc bulge, warding off a full blown pain attack. From this position, try and stand up without moving the spine (use the shoulders and hips). After the initial fragility has resolved, go right back to stage one of the recovery plan in the previous chapters and progress through the stages once again. Generally, you will find that you will recover faster than before.

Does diet factor into back pain?

Some people claim that back pain can be caused by certain diets and foods. I myself have not been able to confirm diet as a major cause. For example, I have heard that eating spicy foods will irritate the gut causing poor abdominal muscle activation, ultimately leading to pain. Yet when discussing training programs with some of the great weightlifting teams from Eastern Europe, they revealed that they purposefully eat a spicy meal prior to Olympic and world competitions to "charge up" their explosive power. It does, however, remain conceivable that for some, bowel irritation could inhibit muscle activation or change posture for exertion.

Do you have tips for relaxing?

What is a relaxing activity for you? If it is walking, try and walk without tension, except for a mild stiffening of the abdominal muscles. Enjoy swinging the arms in a jaunty relaxed manner. If your activity of choice is reading or watching the TV, avoid sitting on a floppy couch—this will force your spine into flexion, causing more pain. You need a firm chair with lumbar support. If reading, place the book on a level higher than your lap or low table, to reduce the tendency to flex the neck and look down. If reading in bed, be very aware of your spine and neck posture – do not let the lumbar spine flatten to the mattress or allow pillows to flex your neck forward. Spare your back – relaxing is a time to let your spine recover!

What about sex?

Ah! You thought we would never get here! During a consultation, when I explain the notion of spine vs. hip motion, I sometime use a visual of the "midnight movement", "the act", coitus! Many patients then exclaim, "Is that why sex is so painful?" Simply bringing awareness to the idea spine motion causes pain is very enlightening for many. Of course, the alternate strategy is to bend about the hips. Regardless of strategy, the old adage, "if it hurts, you're doing it wrong" might be appropriate here. The trick is to find a position that doesn't cause pain and doesn't compromise the natural curves of the spine.

There are some who will argue that the spine is made to move and that this should be trained and encouraged. To these individuals, I respond with the following demonstration to quickly prove to them that this is a myth. I have them place a loaded bar on their shoulders and ask them to perform the "midnight movement" (a back and forth "thrust," if you will) centered through the lumbar spine (recall chapter 6) – pain usually develops quickly and I have made my point.

As a basic rule, if, during intercourse, you are in the top position, you must use the hips. If you are in the bottom position, you must support the natural curves of the spine and avoid initiating movement yourself. If your position of choice involves standing up in a canoe – you are my hero!

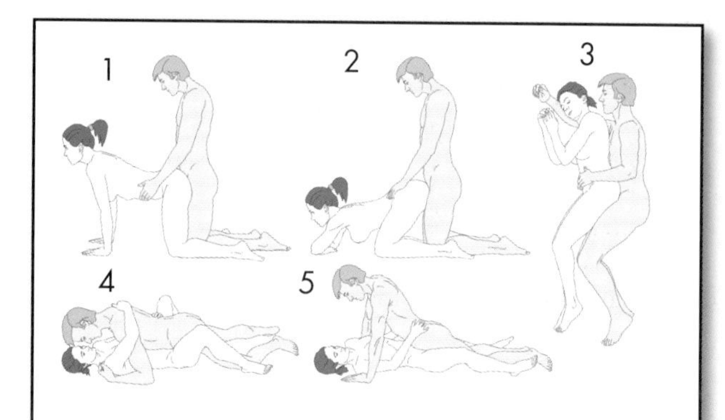

The person on top focusses on hip-hinge motion rather than spine motion. The person on bottom focusses on maintaining a neutral spine. Modify positions to achieve these rules while avoiding individual intolerances. Positions 1 and 2 are best to maintain neutral spine postures. Positions 3 and 4 are more risky and are to be avoided by the flexion and the extension motion intolerant. Position 5 is very difficult to avoid pain in most people.

What about the passive therapies: chiropractic/ massage/PT modalities/traction ?

Passive therapies (having things done to you) are very unlikely to cure your damaged back tissues. These include the PT modalities such as ultrasound and laser therapy. You must be an active participant in your pain management. These therapies may temporarily reduce the pain (or in some cases may increase the pain), but they do not address the cause of your problems. Chiropractors do not fix your back by putting "out of place" bones back into place. This could only be possible if you had a horrible fracture. They can realign collagen fibers that have delaminated to help seal the wall of a disc but must combine this with re-educating movement patterns to remove the movement flaw that caused the collagen to delaminate in the first place. Massage may reduce muscle pain by allowing the muscles to relax, but without postural change the pain will quickly return. No passive approach creates the patterns of movement, the spine stability, and hip mobility needed to remove the tissue stresses that cause pain. If you are working with a practitioner, be sure that they are following the "active" principles in this book (see next question).

What about chiropractors?

I am often asked for my opinion on what I think of chiropractors. I have clinicians around the world to whom I refer patients – many are chiropractors. The ones I refer to may only occasionally manipulate a back, but they have many clinical tools in their treatment repertoire, including an appreciation for removing the movement flaws that cause chronic back pain. If you have a chiropractor who recommends regular visits for months with just manipulation, they are not curing you. Studies show that for some patients with acute disc bulges, one to three manipulations may assist in recovery. The fact remains, however, that no scientific evidence exists that supports repeated manipulations as a cure for back pain. Remember that chiropractic manipulation is not putting "something back into place that was out of place". Our investigations have shown that the manipulations have mostly neurological effects that can reduce muscular spasms or sometimes the opposite – create spasms.

You should find a chiropractor who has evolved to provide "active care": they coach you through pain avoidance strategies and appropriate exercise programs. Many of these chiropractors are familiar with our program and approach – ask them if they are aware of our work. The effective chiropractors are excellent at combining soft tissue manual therapy with the approaches in this book and in doing so, produce long-term positive results.

Out of interest: What makes the great athletes so great?

I have been fortunate to assess and work with some of the strongest, fastest, and most elite athletes in the world – Olympians and world champions from a wide array of sports. My answer to this question is that their gifts are varied, but are not in the ways most people think. They may not be the strongest when tested. The fastest men and women are actually the best relaxers. When muscles contract, both force and stiffness are created. The fastest athletes create muscle pulses of high force to initiate movement and then have the ability to relax to allow ultimate limb speed. For them, core stiffness acts as the center of power while their limbs are actually quite loose. Thus, I would say that the best jumpers, throwers, runners, kickers, punchers, golfers, etc. have the gift of ultra quick muscle relaxation following a sharp contraction (up to six times faster than "average" people). Outside of their physical prowess, this ability is actually a neurological gift. Relaxation rate is very hard to train, but not impossible. I do see many instances in my consults where this natural athleticism was ruined by too much weight training with little focus on neurological component training.

Other great athletes have wonderfully tuned elastic systems in their body – again I have seen this compromised with foolish stretching choices. The best stretches "tune" their elastic bodies instead of "stretching them out". Of course, the mental component of athleticism is huge - the will to win, to not give in, to train, etc. Some of the great athletes have exceptional personalities. But in terms of their backs, they may not lift maximum weight to create supreme back strength. The interested reader may want to read my other book *"Ultimate Back Fitness and Performance"* that discusses these topics in detail.

Get rid of back pain in XXX easy steps (you fill in the number)! Ignore this!

For most people this is a false promise. XXX easy steps do not exist but for a very lucky few. You now realize that getting rid of back pain can be complicated. Understanding your personal pain triggers is essential in you avoiding the cause. The exercises that you have adopted under my guidance have enabled you to bear load and move to achieve a full life. Your work has paid off – but it was neither simple nor easy.

Chapter 17
In Conclusion

In Conclusion

So there you have it! Your owner's manual to your spine. My hope for each and every one of you is that you now have a much more complete and accurate understanding of your back, of these mysterious aggravators we call "triggers," and of the steps and exercises that will allow you to reclaim your life pain-free. You should now have the capability to write your own recovery program that includes conscious efforts to adjust your daily movement patterns as well as a realistic repertoire of rehabilitative exercises.

It is often helpful to keep a journal or notebook during your recovery, not to record your pain levels, but rather your daily activities so that you can look back and review what you have done the day before and take note of whether it made you feel better or worse. Remember that recovery is about finding a balance. If you lose motivation, slip back into old habits and neglect your exercise program, you cannot expect to improve. Contrarily, if you are overambitious and push yourself too hard on days you are pain-free, your body will alert you that it simply wasn't ready by returning to a painful state the next day. Stay motivated, stay realistic, and I am confident that you too can experience the kind of turn-around my patients write me about on a daily basis!

As mentioned previously, this book was written to be consumed by anyone. For those of you with inclinations towards high-performance athletics or an interest in more in-depth back medicine, I would direct you towards my other two books entitled, *"Low Back Disorders: Evidence based prevention and rehabilitation"*, and *"Ultimate Back Fitness and Performance"*. For the rest of you, you should now be equipped with everything you need! Remember that if you return to seek guidance from a qualified physician during your recovery, I would advise you to bring this book with you so that they can familiarize themselves with my work and that you can ensure you are "speaking the same language." The fact remains, that a patient equipped with information is always their own best advocate!

As the Back Mechanic torch has now been passed on to you the reader, I cannot wait to begin to hear your various success stories. Whether it's getting back to the driving range, or being able to crawl into the blanket fort with your kids, or just being able to reach your feet and tie your shoes again, relish these accomplishments! Congratulate yourself on your dedication; you are now reaping the rewards!

Thank you for choosing to go through this rehabilitative journey with me. I would just ask you to promise me one thing, as you continue to reclaim your pain-free life, don't forget to smile!

Glossary

Antalgia: A loss of the normal spine curve due to spine injury or pathology. Antalgia often appears as a "kink" in the spine. Flexion antalgia of the lumbar spine is common with disc bulges – here the spine will have a local flexion curve. Lateral antalgia is also common with acute low back pain caused by a disc.

Compression: Loads applied down the length of the spine cause compression. These could be from muscle forces or from loads applied to the body.

Distal: The lumbar spine is used as the reference baseline for the body in that all other parts are distal from the lumbar spine. The elbow is distal to the shoulder etc.

Kyphosis: The name of the curve of the thoracic spine (those vertebrae connected to a rib). Accentuated curvature associated with a slouched posture or aging is call hyperkyphosis.

Lordosis: The name of the normal curve in the low back. A loss of the curve is hypolordosis and an accentuated curve is called hyperlordosis.

Neural tension: Tight nerves are caused by materials impinging on them somewhere along their length. This causes the nerves to tighten at certain parts, usually causing pain, known as neural tension. This is often confused with what is perceived as tight muscles.

Neutral Spine: This is the shape of a normal spine when standing upright (unless there is a postural deformity). This is the position where the spine is most relaxed and free of joint tensions that are created as the joints are bent away from neutral.

Proximal: The lumbar spine is used as the reference baseline for the body in that it is the most proximal of all other parts. Thus the shoulder is proximal to the elbow.

Shear: The shear axis is perpendicular to the compressive axis (see compression). Shear forces on the spine joints can result from muscle forces and loads applied to or by the body.

Stiffness: Stiffness, while often is a negative term, is essential for a healthy spine as stiffness from muscles allows it to bear load without buckling. Stiffness is also needed in the spine and torso to allow efficient movement in the arms and legs. Stiffness arrests micro-movements of the spine joints to eliminate some types of pain.

Torque (Moment): This refers to a rotational force, for example, a muscle attaching to a bone creates a torque about the joint. Torque enables joints to support static loads and move body segments that make the linkage move.

MOVEMENTS

Flexion: When standing upright and relaxed, the spine is bent forward – this is flexion. Sitting and gardening are activities that cause spine flexion.

Extension: Bending backwards from neutral is an extension movement. This occurs during overhead reaches.

Bending: Moving the spine away from neutral in any direction is bending. This is akin to bending a tree branch in that stresses are developed in the spine.

MUSCLES

Erector Spinae: All spine extensor muscles are collectively known as erector spinae

Gluteus maximus: The major gluteal muscle that primarily externally rotates and extends the hip. The lower portion is most active in the deep squat while the upper portion is more active during walking, running and changing direction.

Gluteus medius: The high and lateral gluteal muscle essential for walking and running, and supporting the pelvis as a level platform for the spine.

Gluteal muscles: All of the gluteal muscles that form the buttocks

Latissimus Dorsi: This important spine stabilizer, and extensor is the major brachiating muscle connecting the upper arm with the torso. This allows all pulling activities, positions the spine to bear load in a safer manner, and enhances abilities needed for daily living.

Multifidus: Made of small slips of muscle that can span a single spine joint level or two or three levels. These slips are responsible for movement control at single joints and are spine extensors.

Oblique muscles: The external and internal oblique muscles are layered with transverse abdominis to form the abdominal wall. They stiffen the core or torso, add stability to the spine, enable twisting motions, and store elastic energy for activities like throwing and hitting a golf ball. They are essential muscles for nearly all activities of daily living.

Rectus Abdominis: The "Six-pack" muscle at the front of the abdomen. It forms an anchor for several abdominal muscles making it important for spine stiffness. It is also a flexor of the torso.

Quadratus lumborum: This muscle runs beside the lumbar spine attaching to every vertebra. It is active during every load bearing activity as it is the major guy wire system of the spine to stiffen the column necessary to bear load.

Index

S

T

V

W

Y

Appendix

Activity Log and Exercise Log

Pain and Activity Ability

Establishing a positive weekly reduction in symptoms is essential. You will forget how you felt a month ago. This log will help you "keep score" of your progress.

ACTIVITY	WEEK									
	1		2		3		4		5	
	YES	NO	YES	NO	YES	NO	YES	NO	YES	NO
I had pain-free periods this week										
I can walk XX minutes before pain begins (list minutes)										
I can sit for XX minutes before pain begins (list minutes)										
I had back pain in bed										
I had back pain when rolling over in bed										
I can pick up 20 pounds off a chair seat without pain										
Activities that are now pain-free (name them)										
Activity 1										
Activity 2										
Activity 3										
Activity 4										
Activity 5										
Activity 6										
Activity 7										

Exercise Log

ACTIVITY		WEEK									
		1	2	3	4	5	6	7	8	9	10
Walking 3 times per day (walking time)	1st										
	2nd										
	3rd										
Modified Curl-up (10 sec holds) (eg 6-4-2 reps)											
Side Plank (10 sec holds) (note the form)											
Birddog (10 sec holds (form and sets/reps)											
Other exercises:	Cat/camel										
	Push (countertop pushups, floor pushups)										
	Pullups (TRX pulls, pullups)										
Add your exercises here:											

Exercise Log Sample: Martina Backstrom

ACTIVITY		WEEK									
		1	2	3	4	5	6	7	8	9	10
Walking 3 times per day (walking time)	1st	15 min									
	2nd	10 min									
	3rd	10 min									
Modified Curl-up (10 sec holds) (eg 6-4-2 reps)		2, 2, 2									
Side Plank (10 sec holds) (note the form)		2, 2, 2									
Birddog (10 sec holds (form and sets/reps)		3, 3, 2									
Other exercises:	Cat/camel	5 reps									
	Push (countertop pushups, floor pushups)	3, 3, 2									
	Pullups (TRX pulls, pullups)	2, 2, 2									
Add your exercises here:											

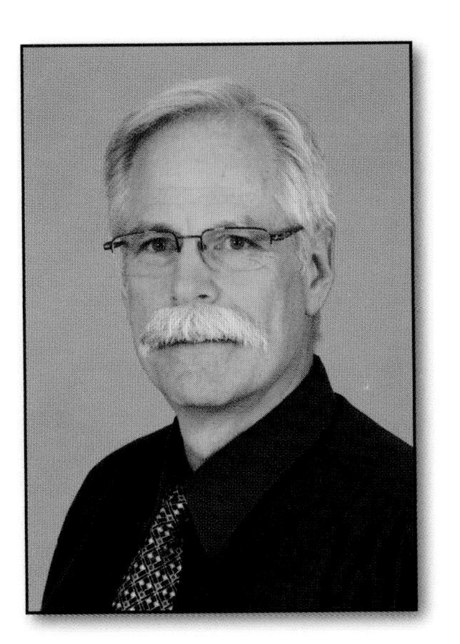

More from Stuart McGill

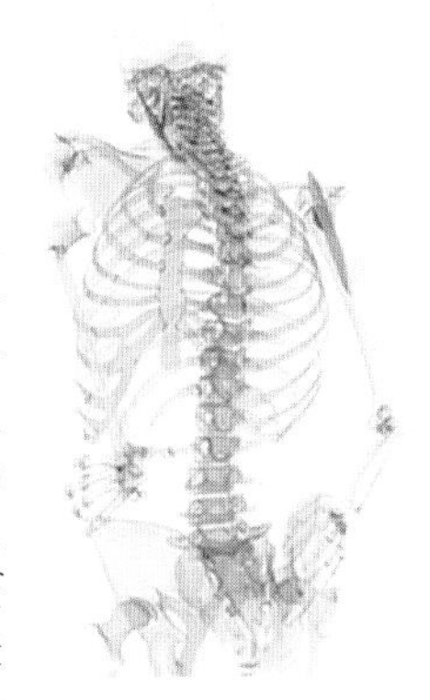

Stuart McGill is a Professor Emeritus (Spine Biomechanics, University of Waterloo). For 32 years he directed laboratory investigations that explored low back function, injury prevention and rehabilitation, and performance training. The new findings were then tested in the clinic. This collective work resulted in over 400 scientific publications that include 4 textbooks. The first book, *"Low Back Disorders: Evidence based prevention and rehabilitation"* (Third edition) was written for clinicians to guide their decision process when prescribing prevention and rehabilitation approaches. Another textbook, *"Ultimate Back Fitness and Performance"* (fifth edition) was written for trainers, coaches, athletes and those interested in enhancing performance of their back while minimizing any loss of resilience. Recently *"The gift of Injury"*, co-written with Champion power lifter Brian Carroll guides the strength athlete out of pain to regaining strength. He completed the knowledge transfer process with the current book, "Back Mechanic" which targeted the lay public with back pain. Collectively this work has received numerous scientific awards. As a consultant, he sees particularly difficult back pain patients and also provides expertise on assessment and reduction of the risk of low back injury to various government agencies, many corporations and legal firms and elite athletes and teams from many countries. His books and technique videos can be seen at www.backfitpro.com

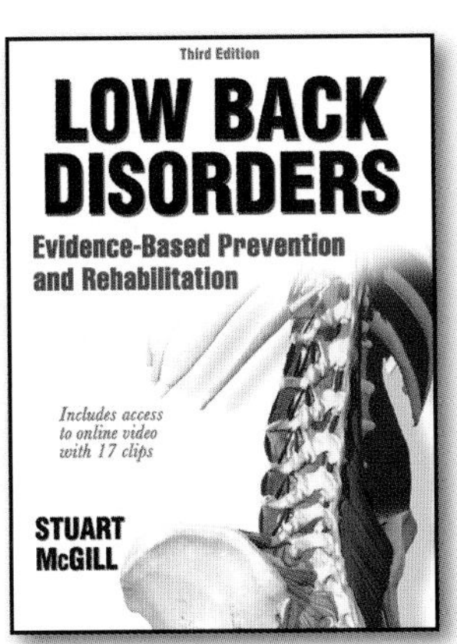

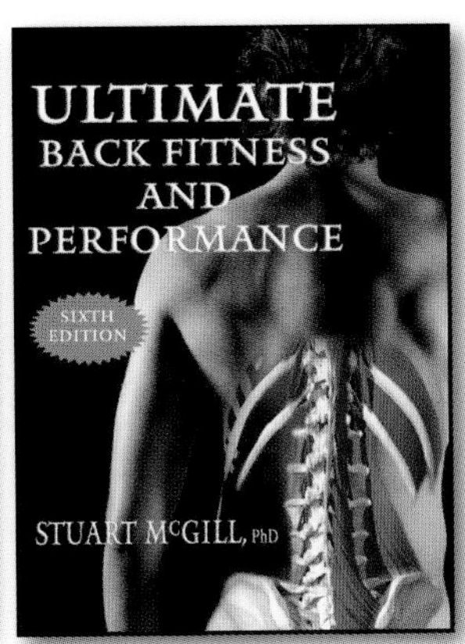

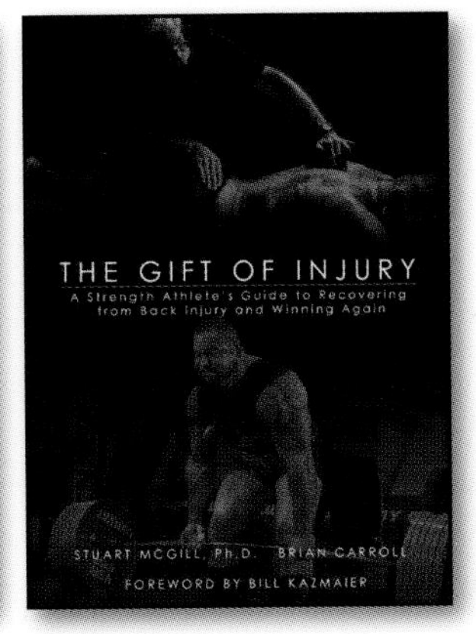

Textbooks

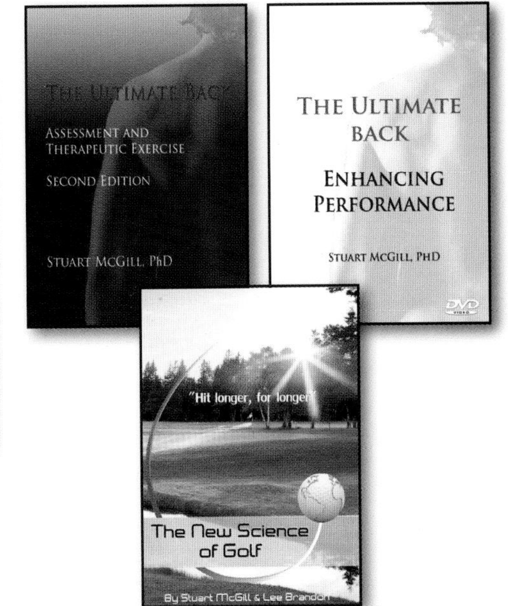

Videos

Notes